THE HAIR-LOSS CURE

THE HAIR-LOSS CURE

A SELF-HELP GUIDE

Find the Cause
Choose the Right Treatment
Monitor Improvement
Cope With Emotional Effects

DAVID H. KINGSLEY, PHD

iUniverse, Inc.
New York Bloomington

THE HAIR-LOSS CURE
A SELF-HELP GUIDE

The information, ideas, and suggestions in this book are not intended as a substitute for professional medical advice. Before following any suggestions contained in this book, you should consult your personal physician. Neither the author nor the publisher shall be liable or responsible for any loss or damage allegedly arising as a consequence of your use or application of any information or suggestions in this book.

iUniverse books may be ordered through booksellers or by contacting:

iUniverse
1663 Liberty Drive
Bloomington, IN 47403
www.iuniverse.com
1-800-Authors (1-800-288-4677)

Because of the dynamic nature of the Internet, any Web addresses or links contained in this book may have changed since publication and may no longer be valid. The views expressed in this work are solely those of the author and do not necessarily reflect the views of the publisher, and the publisher hereby disclaims any responsibility for them.

ISBN: 978-1-935278-04-7 (pbk)
ISBN: 978-1-935278-05-4 (ebk)

Printed in the United States of America

iUniverse rev. date: 1/26/09

To my wife, Yvonne

CONTENTS

ACKNOWLEDGMENTS

I am deeply indebted to my mother, Betty, for her constant encouragement; to my stepfather, Tony; to my sisters, Susan and Helen; and my mother-in-law, Sarah.

Recognition is also due to my father, without whom I wouldn't have become a trichologist; and to Dr. Hugh Rushton, Dr. Michael Norris, and Dr. Jane Portlock without whom I wouldn't have attained my PhD.

Thanks are also due to Maureen and Gordon Burnett, Mike and Mary Caravaglio, Mo, Sebastian, Caroline, James, and Jim, whose unquestioning support and encouragement were invaluable.

A special thanks to all my staff at British Science Corporation and my trichology centers for working so hard and freeing up time for me to write this book. Extra special thanks to Michele Como, Denis DaSilva, Lorraine Massey, Steve Jones, Suzanne Ruffo, Dr. Paul Cotterill, and Dr. Cap Lesesne.

Last, but far from least, a huge hug and kisses to Yvonne, without whom none of this would have been possible.

PREFACE

THE HAIR-LOSS CURE

I use the word cure to mean the partial or complete improvement of some hair loss conditions. There could be many reasons why you are losing hair. Some of these causes are only temporary, particularly if they are due to hair breakage, stress, or diet. These types of hair loss conditions can be helped, the hair can be regrown; the hair loss can be cured.

Even with genetic hair loss, there are many treatment options that can help. As I discuss in this book, some treatments may slow down the progression of the condition, some may stabilize it, while others can actually regrow your hair.

I have used many of the treatment regimens described in this book to help my patients' hair. I have also used these treatments for my own hair loss. Here is my story.

MY PERSONAL HAIR STORY

My interest in hair started when I worked at my father's trichology (hair and scalp) center in London, England, during my vacation from high school. I had a full, bushy head of hair that had to be thinned to look reasonably "under control". My girl friend, Yvonne (now my wife), is a cosmetologist, and she kidded me by saying she needed shears to cut my hair!

In 1980, I qualified as a board-certified trichologist (hair and scalp specialist) through the Institute of Trichologists in London and started making appointments to see patients with hair loss. My first consultation was with a woman who was extremely distraught about her severely thinning hair. Although I was able to help her, I was concerned that I wasn't prepared for this level of emotional distress from a patient. At the time, the psychological impact of hair loss wasn't part of the trichology training syllabus or something that was even discussed at college.

Shortly after this my wife and I moved to the United States, and I began to work at my father's trichology business in New York. As time went on, I noticed that a large percentage of men and women who sought my help were exceptionally upset about losing their hair. Many of them said that they had seen other hair-loss specialists who showed no empathy for their condition. As well as treating their hair loss, I also tried to help these patients cope with their condition, but I felt that I needed more knowledge to advise them effectively. Around the same time, my own hair was beginning to thin, but I took little notice.

To learn more, I went back to college part-time and took a degree in psychology at the City University of New York. This extra work, coupled with more job responsibility, increased my stress level and affected the way that I ate. I continued to see more of my scalp, and I began to become quite concerned. My family has a history of hair loss, and my condition looked like a combination of male pattern alopecia (genetic hair loss) and telogen effluvium (excessive hair shedding).

After I graduated, I decided to further enhance my knowledge by enrolling in a doctorate program with the University of Portsmouth in England. It was a part-time course that required me to travel back to England a few times a year. Fortunately, I was able to conduct a great deal of my research, which included studying the psychological impact of hair loss, in New York.

Shortly after I began my PhD course, I started my own trichology center in New York called British Science Corporation. My level of stress became even greater. I was trying to start a business, take care of my family, and work toward my doctorate, all while my own hair loss persisted. I continued helping other people but, ironically, had little or no time to help myself. In fact, I became very self-conscious about my continuing hair loss, particularly as I was a certified hair-loss specialist. I even used a hairpiece for a short period of time.

Once I attained my doctorate, I decided to sort out the factors behind my hair loss condition. I realized that my hair loss wasn't triggered by one thing but by many factors, including family history (genetics), high stress, and a poor diet. I began to treat each of these causes. For the genetic hair loss, I began using an extra strength (5 percent) minoxidil solution, Propecia (the Merck brand), and the HairMax LaserComb (Lexington International), all in combination with my own British Science trichology stimulant treatments. To help reduce my stress, I started working out and doing meditation exercises. For my poor diet I began to eat properly, balancing my diet with smaller, more frequent meals. I began taking a vitamin/mineral supplement that I formulated specifically for hair loss (which I now recommend to my patients), and took Nourkrin (Pharma Medico International), a protein supplement formulated for thinning hair. I also began coloring my hair because a lot of gray hairs were growing in, making my hair appear thinner. In addition, I had a full physical at my physician that included a check of my thyroid (the results of my physical, thankfully, were normal).

After a few months, I began to see a big difference in my hair. I noticed a lot of regrowth, and the amount of hair I was losing slowed down and eventually returned to normal levels. My hair started improving considerably, so much so that I was able to throw away my hairpiece!

I continued to follow these treatment and lifestyle changes and my hair remained in great condition. I then became greedy! I wanted to improve my hair even more. So I decided to have some minor hair-restoration surgery to the front and crown areas of my head (from Dr. Paul Cotterill). Now I am even more satisfied with my hair and even look forward to washing and styling it every day!

The concern over losing my own hair, combined with my clinical experience in helping patients with hair problems and the knowledge that I gleaned from my research on hair loss, has left me with a unique insight into helping you cope with your hair loss; find the causes of your hair loss; and choose the right treatments for your hair loss.

I didn't allow my hair loss to ruin my life and I hope that this book helps prevent your hair loss from ruining yours.

The Hair-Loss Cure: A Self-Help Guide will steer you onto the road to hair recovery!

INTRODUCTION

"Losing my hair has been the most disturbing event of my life."
"Losing my hair has made me depressed."
"I feel undesirable as a result of my hair loss."
"I get no understanding from others about my hair loss."

These are some of the quotes I hear everyday from my patients regarding a condition that effects approximately 60 percent of women and 85 percent of men at some time in their lives: *hair loss*. However slight, hair loss can have a devastating effect on people's lives. It can be the last thing they think about when they go to bed and the first thing they think about when they wake up. It can cause people to change their normal daily routines ("I'm not going out today because it's too windy and people will see my scalp"), or it can take many hours out of their day ("I don't go out until I'm satisfied with the way my hair looks)."

If you are losing excessive amounts of hair, how can it affect your everyday life? How can you find out why it's falling out? How do you treat your hair fall and monitor that the treatment is working? The depth in which *The Hair-Loss Cure: A Self Help Guide* answers these questions makes it a very useful tool to help you cope with your hair loss. In the preface of this book, I briefly describe how the reactions of some of my patients to their hair loss and the concern I had for my own hair loss encouraged me to search for answers to these questions. My quest began in 1980 with my very first patient expressing severe anxiety over losing her hair, and it continued through many years of further education and research. My own hair loss condition was an extra incentive in studying the best ways to treat and cope with losing hair.

Are you really losing hair?

If you see more hair falling out, the first thing that you need to do is ascertain whether you are actually losing your hair or just experiencing normal shedding. This question is discussed in Chapter 1: Are You Really Losing Hair? Not all people who see more hair fall (the amount that comes out in the wash or the comb) are actually experiencing hair thinning (less hair on their scalp). Sometimes seeing more hair loss is normal; it could be a seasonal occurrence or just your regular hair cycle.

How do you cope with hair loss?

Chapter 2: How You Can Cope with Hair Loss, is an unique chapter when compared to other hair-loss books as it discusses many of the psychological effects of hair loss and recommends ways to help you overcome them. The suggestions in this chapter have helped me and many of my patients control some of the very real fears that we experienced as a result of hair loss. *The Hair-Loss Cure: A Self-Help Guide* will help point you in the right direction to regain the control over your life that hair loss often takes away.

What is causing your hair to fall out or to thin?

If you think that you are experiencing hair loss, you need to find all the possible reasons as to why you are losing your hair. You should then find ways to correct the problem. Trying to discover all the factors that have caused your hair to fall out or to thin is often like detective work. You need to search carefully through all the information that you and your doctor have compiled, deciding what is relevant and what can be discarded. Sometimes the answer only appears when you've exhausted all other possibilities.

Chapter 3: Why You Are Losing Hair, explains that hair loss is often not caused by just one factor, but by a combination of two, three, or even more factors simultaneously affecting your hair cycle. Therefore, treatments that are designed for helping one aspect will not always help another. In addition, some treatments that improve the symptoms will not necessarily help the actual causes, leading to occasional relapses or a continued slow deterioration.

In this chapter, I have listed the main causes of hair loss under the heading "7 Hs of Hair Loss". These include: Heredity, Hormones, Health, Hassle (stress), Hunger (diet), Healing (medications), and Hairdressing. I discuss each of the 7Hs at length, so you will be able to judge for yourself which causes are relevant for your hair loss condition.

What treatments are available that may be helpful?

With so many treatments to choose from, how do you know which treatment is right for you? Chapter 4: Treating Your Hair Loss, helps you choose the best treatment for each possible cause of your hair loss.

As many factors may be causing your hair to fall out, you could need many treatments to improve your condition. To minimize the difficulty in deciding on the best treatment, I have clearly discussed each of the treatment options under each heading of the 7Hs. This will help you determine the best type of treatment for whatever factors are causing your hair loss. Depending on what is causing your hair loss, some of these treatments will help you improve or even cure your condition.

How can you tell whether the treatment is working?

Chapter 5: How You Can Monitor Whether the Treatment Is Working, is another unique chapter of this book when compared to other hair-loss books. It will help you take control of your hair loss condition. This chapter will help you examine the progress of any treatments that you decide to use. It will help you measure whether your hair loss is excessive or normal, and it will help you see whether a thinning area is improving or becoming larger.

The Hair-Loss Cure: A Self-Help Guide will also help you to measure the extent that your hair loss is affecting your usual daily activities. If you find that it is, this book will help you come to terms with your problem and stop it from affecting your daily lifestyle.

The final chapter, The Bottom Line, sums up the book and concisely brings all the advice together. The Appendix discusses hair-loss conditions further and in depth for those who wish to learn more. References and Further Reading will help you find Websites, books, and medical journals to help improve your understanding about your hair loss condition.

The Hair-Loss Cure: A Self-Help Guide will help your hair—and it will help *you.*

ONE

ARE YOU REALLY LOSING HAIR?

"When I started to lose my hair, I took a few of my best friends into my confidence. They just brushed it off and said 'It doesn't look like you're losing hair, so don't worry.'" Nigel, twenty-eight-year-old registered nurse.

"My husband looks at my hair and can't understand why I'm so worried. He says that it looks the same to him and that he wishes he had half of what I have!" Monica, thirty-five-year-old housewife.

Is Nigel really losing his hair, or are his friends correct? Is Monica's husband right to not take her concerns seriously? How do you know whether your hair is falling out excessively or whether it's normal and nothing to worry about?

Most people at some time in their lives notice more hair in the sink, on the pillow, or in the comb. If this happens to you, should you worry? Is this the first sign of hair loss? Does it mean that you are going bald?

Usually, most people quickly become aware of their own hair loss; they see more hair shedding or they see more of their scalp or both. Hair shedding is the amount of hair that falls out during your normal daily lifestyle, such as by combing, brushing, or washing your hair. Hair thinning is less hair density in a particular area of the scalp, such as a wider parting or a receding hairline. Although hair thinning can occur without any obvious excessive hair shedding, it most often occurs if your hair sheds excessively for a long period of time. For instance, Mike, a twenty-three-year-old construction worker, first noticed hair on his pillow. His shower didn't have a "catch" so he never saw loss while washing his hair. At first he thought nothing of it, but then he started seeing hair all over the place—on the bathroom floor and even in his food! Within a few weeks he noticed that his hair had thinned in the front and had receded a little at his temples.

CAN I HAVE HAIR THINNING WITHOUT EXCESSIVE SHEDDING?

Thinning hair is often, but not always, the result of excessive hair shedding. For example, Barbara, a thirty-three-year-old music store manager, was astonished to see the back of her head in a mirror at a local restaurant. "I first noticed my hair loss when I was sitting in a restaurant. It was raining, so I got drenched on the way; and I saw my scalp in one of the mirrors. It was very upsetting for me." While waiting for her friends to arrive, she noticed that she could see through her hair, right down to the crown of her scalp. Usually her hair was carefully blow-dried and styled, but due to the rain, her wet hair hung limp and exposed the thinning area. It was a shock for Barbara because she hadn't noticed any of the common warning signs, such as excessive hair shedding, before she saw that her hair had thinned. Although her hair had likely been thinning for some time before she noticed, the lack of excessive hair in the brush kept it from her attention. It crept up on her without warning.

DO I HAVE EXCESSIVE HAIR FALL?

What Is the Number for Average Daily Hair Fall?

The average number of hair that most people should expect to lose each day is between forty and one hundred twenty hairs. Why the discrepancy? It's mainly because of the difference in the amount of hair people have on their heads, as well as the difference in the length of time the hair remains in its growing phase (see the Appendix for how the average daily hair fall is calculated).

How Many Hairs Do I Have on My Head?

We are born with all of our hair follicles; none are produced after birth. The follicles are usually found in groups of two to four hairs that are spaced at intervals. The average person has approximately 80,000 to 150,000 hairs on his or her head, depending on hair type and natural hair color (overall, the average is 100,000). If you have blonde hair, you tend naturally to have a higher number of hairs on your head because the hair fiber s are very fine and more strands per square inch are able to "fit." If you have red hair, you tend naturally to have a lower number of hairs because your individual hair fiber s are coarser and allow for fewer hairs per square inch on your scalp.

Fine hairs are usually straight and limp, with little natural body; coarser hairs are usually curlier, with a lot of natural body. Under a microscope, the cross section (looking at the cut end of a hair fiber, straight on) of a fine, straight hair strand is round in shape. The cross section of a medium-textured, wavy hair strand is oval. The cross section of a coarse, curly hair strand is an elliptical shape.

- People with coarse, curly hair usually average about 80,000 hairs.
- People with medium, wavy hair usually average about 100,000 hairs.
- People with fine, straight hair often have 120,000 to 150,000 hairs.

For How Long Does My Hair Grow?

The hair cycle consists of many phases (see the Appendix). The growing phase (called *anagen*) is the most relevant time to ascertain hair length. This phase of the hair cycle lasts for about one thousand days (three years). The hair grows at an average speed of a half-inch per month (or six inches per year); therefore, the average length an individual hair strand grows is approximately eighteen inches. Some people's growing phases are much longer (more than five years), and some are much shorter (less than two years). This means that some people can grow their hair down to their feet, while others cannot grow it beyond their shoulders.

Why Is There Such a Large Difference Between the Amounts of Hair a Person Should Lose Every Day?

Although the average amount of hair on a person's head is approximately 100,000 strands, not everyone has exactly this amount. Moreover, not everyone's hair cycle is three years. For instance, the small percentage of people who can grow their hair down to their feet may have a five-to ten-year hair cycle! Some people only have a two-year cycle, so they are unable to grow their hair beyond their shoulders. This explains that different people can and will have vastly different normal hair fall amounts. Also, remember that forty to one hundred twenty hairs are only an average. Some people will naturally see more than one hundred twenty hairs fall out, while others will see fewer than forty. In addition, if your average is one hundred, you will not lose one hundred hairs every day. Some days you may find very few hairs; other days you may find lots more hair. So don't panic if you see more hairs coming out, as long as you see less on other days.

Can Hair Loss Amounts in the Average Range Be Too Much?

Hair loss amounts in the "average" range can sometimes still be excessive. If you count your hair over a few weeks and notice that about an average of ninety hairs fall out, you might decide that this is okay because it fits nicely in the "normal" range. However, if you were only losing, say, forty-five hairs per day when you were washing before, ninety is *twice* as many hairs as *your* normal average. This could mean that you have excessive hair loss. Therefore, it is important that you only compare your hair fall with your own history, not with another person's hair history.

Can Hair Loss Amounts That Are More Than the Average Range Be Okay?

Hair loss amounts higher than the "average" can be normal. If you count ninety hairs as an average and you're only used to seeing forty-five, you would probably become concerned. However, you need to ask yourself, "When did I previously wash my hair?" If you used to wash your hair every day and noticed about forty-five hairs falling out but recently skipped a day or two between washes, then seeing ninety hairs could be normal. The reason for this is that hair loss accumulates; the less often you wash your hair, the more hair fall you see when you do wash it. Therefore, the forty-five hairs that you lost on a daily wash basis will accumulate to ninety if you wash every two days, one hundred thirty-five if you wash every three days, and so on. I had a patient who hadn't washed his hair for three months! Every time he washed his hair, he saw it fall out, and so he washed it less. The problem was that when he *did* decide to wash it, weeks of normal hair loss had accumulated and this compounded the problem. Once I explained to him that his normal hair loss was mounting up between washes, he began washing his hair more often. As he began to see less coming out, he felt confident in washing more frequently.

Clearly the old wives' tale that says washing your hair makes it fall out more is incorrect! Wash your hair as often as you want. Any hair that comes out has already been released by the follicle and so is ready to fall. By not washing your hair, you allow this normal hair amount to build up. Therefore, when you do wash it, it looks like more is falling out, making you needlessly worried about losing hair.

Is Washing the Only Place to Look for Excessive Hair Loss?

You can also see excessive hair loss during different styling processes, such as in the comb or brush, or even on the pillow in the morning. Some people see hair everywhere—on their shoulders, on the kitchen or bathroom floor, even on their spouses' clothes. Although you may see one hundred hairs when you wash, you probably lose about 20 percent more (one hundred twenty total) during the day. This is due to hair styling or just the result of gravity.

Could My Hair Loss Just Be Seasonal?

Many people ask me if they should expect to see more hair loss in the autumn. Unlike most animals with hair, humans do not have seasonal molting, although some people do seem to experience more hair loss at certain times of the year. We don't molt because most of our hair follicles have independent cycles from their neighboring follicles. One hair on your head could be in its growing phase, while the hair next door could be in its resting phase. Therefore, if you see more hair fall in the autumn, you need to ask yourself, "Do I have extra hair loss at this time most years?" If the answer is yes, then you may have seasonal hair loss; if the answer is no, you should consider seeing a specialist.

Is My Hair Loss Just Breakage?

Seeing more hair coming out can often be due to breakage from changing your styling technique, being careless when brushing or combing, or the result of a bad chemical process. Also, if your hair is thinning, those finer, thinner hairs can be more susceptible to breakage. One way to tell whether the hair is breaking or falling from the root is to look at the root end of the fiber. If you see a "bulb," then it has probably come from the root; if not, then it may well be breakage. If the hair has already fallen and you are unsure which is the root end, gently move your fingers down the strand of hair. One way will feel smooth, the other will feel rough. The root should be toward the rougher end.

You can also sometimes tell whether the hair is breaking by looking at your scalp. If you see lots of stubble, then it may be breakage. Although breakage is not hair loss per se, it can still cause thinning and be very worrisome. This is why I always include breakage as a form of hair loss and treat it with similar seriousness.

Is My Hair Length Important when Assessing Hair Loss?

Length of hair can be very important in assessing excessive loss. The longer your hair, the more you will see when it falls out because there is more of it in bulk. For instance, if your hair is six inches long and twenty hairs fall out, the quantity lost will seem greater than fifty hairs that are only one inch long. That doesn't mean that you are losing more hair. In fact, some of the patients I have seen only noticed their hair falling out after they grew their hair longer.

It is important, therefore, to look at the number of hairs that have fallen out, not the bulk quantity in your hand. The only time that the bulk quantity is relevant is if your hair length has more or less stayed the same and you are seeing more in your hand.

IS MY HAIR THINNING?

Most people's hair becomes thinner as they get older. Just as your skin changes, often leading to wrinkles, so your hair follicles become smaller, producing a slightly shorter, finer hair. If enough finer hairs are produced then more space between them develops, causing a thinner look. In this case you can have the same number of hairs as before, but because they are finer in texture, your hair will look thinner. An analogy is with a forest. In the summer, the trees are in full bloom and it is difficult to see through them. In the winter, the fallen leaves give an appearance of "thinner" trees and allow you to see through the forest more easily. The numbers of trees are the same, but the forest has a totally different look.

Another way that your hair can look thinner is if you've lost excessive amounts of hair that do not grow back or take a long time to grow back.

How Can I Tell Whether My Hair Is Thinning?

As mentioned earlier, there are two ways your hair can look thinner. The obvious one is that your partings look wider due to two causes: more space between each hair fiber because the strand is becoming finer, or fewer hairs in number on your head.

The usual places for the hair to look thinner are on the crown of your scalp, the frontal hairline, and in the middle of your scalp (the area between the frontal hairline and the crown of your head). When you part your hair, more space than there used to be may indicate that your hair is thinning.

Thinning may also occur at your temples (also called *recession*), or it may occur in a diffuse manner, which means that it is evenly spread over the entire scalp. In addition, there can be circular areas that are devoid of hair and feel smooth or stubbly.

A slightly different version of hair thinning that I often see is one where the ponytail is thinner; that is, you can wrap a band around the hair of your ponytail more times than you could previously. Often, your partings are similar in density to what they were previously. This could mean that your hair is breaking more, or it could mean that more long hair is falling out than is being replaced by regrowing shorter hair (a condition called *telogen effluvium*, which is discussed in the Appendix).

Different types of hair thinning or thinning in different areas of your scalp can indicate that a different factor is causing your hair loss. Thus, it is important to have an expert examine your condition to identify which type of hair loss you have (see Chapter 3 and the Appendix for more information).

Can the Look of the Scalp Indicate Hair Loss?

Some hair-loss conditions may be accompanied with an oilier or flakier scalp. This does not mean that you will necessarily see more hair coming out or that the scalp condition is causing the loss. The change in the scalp comes about because genetic hair loss is often the result of increased sensitivity to male hormones in the follicle; this can also lead to the sebaceous or oil glands becoming larger and more active, resulting in a greasier scalp. Some flaky scalp conditions are aggravated by increased scalp oil, so it is quite common for the scalp to flake or look oilier with this hair loss condition. However, mild flaking does not usually cause the hair to fall out nor does the hair loss make the scalp flaky. They are just the result of the same trigger mechanism.

Occasionally, the scalp can have acne-looking lesions or red patches. It may appear smooth or, if you gently pinch the skin, look like the skin of an onion. Some of these scalp conditions may be relevant in assessing the cause of your hair loss, as they could indicate a scarring type of hair loss (*cicatricial alopecia*) or *alopecia areata* (see the Appendix for more information).

If you have a scalp problem or are unsure if your scalp condition is causing hair loss, I suggest you see a specialist.

MY HAIR IS FALLING OUT OR THINNING, WHAT SHOULD I DO?

If you have ascertained that your hair is either falling out excessively or thinning you are probably very concerned. You may even be finding that your hair loss is beginning to affect your quality of life—what you eat, how often you go out, how you feel about yourself, and so on. You could be changing your daily routine to compensate for your thinner hair. You may go out less or take longer to be satisfied with the way your hair looks. You may even feel that the problem has made you more stressed and anxious, possibly affecting your work and family life.

In the next chapter, you will learn how to cope with losing your hair so that it doesn't affect your daily life. This chapter not only combines my own experiences with worries that my patients have had, but also encompasses a lot of research into the effects of hair loss on quality of life. This chapter will give you advice on how best to overcome your hair loss fears, and will help you live your life as you did before you noticed your hair loss.

TWO

HOW YOU CAN COPE WITH HAIR LOSS

So what is it about hair that causes such concern when it falls out and such joy when it is styled just right? What makes it so easy to use as the butt of a joke? I recall seeing a film when I was a teenager where two women were fighting over some money and one pulled the other's hair, which came off in her hand. After a split second, in which it took the audience to realize it was a wig, everyone in the theater broke out in hysterical laughter. Would you have also laughed? If your friend or spouse laughed, does it mean that he or she is insensitive to your hair loss?

I remember a young man in his early twenties with thinning hair being the brunt of jokes from friends and families. Is this an example of playfulness or insensitivity? The giving and taking of mild teasing is something most of us do with our friends and relatives. It's part of the fabric of friendship and camaraderie. However, is hair loss fodder for gentle teasing? Would you tease your friend's acne or the scar your sister got from a fall or the birthmark on your brother's face? Are these even fair comparisons? Some people who are losing their hair would say, categorically, *yes*. "Unless someone is experiencing hair loss, they could never truly understand what it's like," says Bob, a twenty-eight-year-old garage mechanic.

THE PSYCHOLOGICAL EFFECTS OF HAIR LOSS

Hair, though mildly useful for protecting our heads, has an important social and decorative role. Since Samson and Delilah were dating in biblical times, hair has symbolized strength, masculinity, and virility for men and beauty and fertility for women. This is borne out by the fact that every year people spend billions of dollars on shampoos, conditioners, styling agents, and treatments that claim to regrow hair. Hair is often the first thing you notice when meeting someone and it is usually the last thing you fuss with before a social event or business meeting. By changing its shape with a setting gel, its color with highlights, or its style with a new haircut, you are able to considerably alter your features and your appearance. No wonder why losing hair can cause stress and anxiety and affect a person's body image and self-esteem.

So what are the specific psychological effects of hair loss? There have been many studies in this area, including part of my PhD thesis (see References and Further Reading), and the results indicate that losing your hair may change your everyday quality of life in some of the following ways.

Anxiety/Depression

Many people with hair loss become very anxious and depressed. Sometimes people experience feelings of despair (exasperation that their hair will not stop falling out), sadness, worry, apprehension, anger at their condition, and fear of going bald. In addition to becoming very stressed, some hair-loss sufferers develop panic attacks.

Lack of Self Esteem

People with hair loss often become dissatisfied with their body image and view themselves differently than how they did before. Many feel embarrassed about losing their hair and unattractive to others—even their spouses and friends—because their hair is thinning. They also feel that other people are always looking at their thinning hair, making them feel even more uncomfortable about their appearance.

Social Problems

Frequently, people with hair loss tend to socialize or date less. They feel that because they are less attractive, there is little point dating. They turn down advances of others because if they get too close, the other person will notice their hair thinning and be turned off. Even married people, or ones in long-term relationships, with hair loss are afraid that their husband, wife, or partner will notice that they are losing hair and stop loving them as a result. Some of my patients don't want their spouse or partner to know that they are seeing me for hair loss because of this fear.

In addition, some people with thinning hair take much longer to get ready to go out because they are trying to hide their scalp. Some may decide that it's not worth taking the time in the first place.

Lack of Support

People without hair loss often cannot see what all the fuss is about, so when a friend or spouse begins to lose his or her hair, they appear aloof and uncaring. As a result, the people who are losing hair feel that their friends and families are failing to be supportive. This usually happens when the hair first begins to fall out and thinning is not yet noticeable.

Sometimes, they are not taken seriously when they see a physician about their hair loss, thus adding to the problem. Many physicians don't realize the psychological impact caused by hair loss and so take the concerns of a patient losing his or her hair less seriously than they should.

Loss Of Control

As there is no treatment that can stop hair loss instantly, people losing their hair occasionally feel that they are unable to control their condition. Over time, this feeling worsens and begins to affect the way they feel about their lives overall.

OVERCOMING SOME OF THE PSYCHOLOGICAL EFFECTS OF HAIR LOSS

If your life has been affected in some or all of the ways listed previously, how can you overcome your fears and get back to living a normal life?

The first thing I want to stress is that if your hair loss worries are truly changing the way you live your life, seek help from a psychologist or psychiatrist who understands the issues you are experiencing.

If you are finding that your hair loss is affecting your quality of life in only a small way, the following section may help you overcome your concerns. I have listed the most common concerns from men and women that I have heard over the years, along with my suggestions for how they might cope with their hair loss. I'm sure there are many more—some that you may have that I haven't mentioned—but I've tried to address the most frequently stated ones. They are not in any particular order. Some of my suggestions may be difficult for you to hear, but I feel that they will help guide you in the right direction.

"I'm frightened to wash my hair."

For many people, hair-wash days are the worst days of the week; this is when they see lots of hair falling out. People dread having to wash their hair but know it is necessary because their hair is starting to look dirty and their scalp is itchy.

Most hair that you see lost during the wash stopped growing approximately six to sixteen weeks before. The less the hair is washed, the more hair loss accumulates. So don't be afraid to wash your hair. In fact, wash it as frequently as you are able and you'll actually see less hair fall out. In addition, your hair looks best when it is freshly washed and dried. It tends to have more body and shine and will allow you to look your best as you start your day. Don't be afraid to use styling products, colors, or perms, as these will give your hair more body and boost the way you feel about it. Washing hair does *not* cause more hair to fall out.

"I don't want anybody mentioning to me that I have hair loss."

A lot of people cringe if anyone mentions their hair loss to them. The last thing they would want is to be told that their hair has become thin enough for someone else to see. Also, some of my patients have said that they notice other people in their workplace with thinning hair. They want to talk to them about it but hesitate because they aren't sure what their reaction will be.

Although it is often helpful for people to talk about their condition with others, it's best not to approach another person with hair loss unless he or she approaches you first (especially women). Many people don't want to be reminded of their problem or are reluctant to talk about it. In these situations, if you are confident enough, talk in a group about your hair loss and what you're doing to combat it within earshot of the other person. Then see whether he or she approaches you at a later time.

"I'm frightened that my hair isn't growing back."

Often, people with hair loss feel that their hair is not growing back and that they will be bald in a matter of weeks. For most hair-loss conditions, such as genetic hair loss and telogen effluvium (see Appendix for more information on these hair-loss conditions), this is not true. The hair does regrow, although it may go through a longer resting phase. The first things to look for with regrowth are the presence of roots (if you color your hair) or the need for a haircut. Under both these circumstances, you know that the hair that is not falling out is growing.

To see whether there is any new hair, dry your hair after a hair-wash and look along the parting. You will see some shorter hairs, which indicate that new hairs are growing. This means that although you are losing lots of hair, some of it is regrowing (also see Chapter 5, which explains how to measure hair regrowth).

"I collect the hair that falls out in the shower."

It is fine in the short term to monitor daily fluctuations in hair fall. However, on occasion, I have seen patients who have collected their hair for many months or years and have kept them all! When they come to see me, they literally bring in carrier bags full of hair they have collected.

I suggest to these people to do a hair count (see Chapter 5) and then dispose of the hair. They do not need past visual reminders that their hair was falling out excessively; they can see by today's wash whether it is still falling out. If you are counting, make sure to do it only infrequently (every two weeks or monthly), as the hair loss amounts will not change rapidly on a daily basis. Also, only count the wash hairs. Do not try to count every hair that you lose, as it's impractical to collect all the hairs from your pillow, clothing, and so on.

"I'm constantly running my hands through my hair."

Many of my patients continually run their hands through their hair to see whether it is still falling out and, if it is, by how much. This action can become obsessive, with someone looking for how much hair is coming out literally hundreds of times a day.

Hair loss amounts don't change that rapidly, so continuous pulling on the hair will not accurately indicate whether the hair loss is improving or worsening. Also, I find that if a person pulls on his or her hair and does not see any hair the first time, he or she will repeat the action four or five times until hair comes out. It is almost as if people want continuous proof that their hair is falling out.

If you find yourself doing this, try to become more aware of the action. It can be habitual, and so you may find that you don't realize you're doing it. Then find something to make your hands become active, such as typing on the computer, to try and slowly break the habit.

"Friends and family don't take my hair loss seriously and underestimate its importance to me."

It can be frustrating for a person with hair loss to hear "It doesn't look bad" or "I don't know what you're talking about" or "There are worse things in life than losing your hair." Hair loss is relative to how you feel about it. Just because you're not bald doesn't mean you don't have hair loss. Just because you hide the condition well doesn't mean a problem doesn't exist. Don't feel guilty. If you're worried that your hair is thinning and your friends or family don't seem to be supportive, don't let that stop you from finding out how to help the problem.

Some people feel that talking to friends from an Internet chat room that deals with hair loss can help them feel more supported than talking to their families. The Internet also has the advantage of anonymity, so people in the chat room cannot physically see your condition (unless you send a photo). I have found this to be very helpful for some people and a great way to find out what other hair loss sufferers are going through. However, some sites are more orientated toward selling their products, so beware.

"Friends and family just complain about all the money I've spent."

They spend money at the hairdresser or barber and on make-up or after-shave. It is important for you to look the best you can look. Obviously, you don't want to waste money on a magical hair cure, so it's up to you to make sure that you thoroughly research the treatment regimen that you are being advised to follow. Don't feel that you must make a decision immediately. Give yourself time to go home, and either discuss it with someone who is supportive or think about it yourself. Moreover, if you do follow a particular program, make sure that you give it at least three months to work.

"I feel that other people are always staring at my hair."

Many people with hair loss feel that others are always looking at their thin spots or staring at their hair. This can make them feel very self-conscious and, in extreme cases, stop them from socializing at all.

I have studied this in depth and have found that this is not happening as much as you think—that is, people are probably not looking at your hair. Think back before you had hair loss. Were you looking at everyone else's hair to see whether it was thinning? Probably not. If you don't have a particular problem, then it wouldn't occur to you to look for it in another person. The person you think is looking at your hair may just be looking at you because you are conversing or because he or she likes the way you look.

When you socialize you are about three or four feet apart from the person to whom you are talking. Remember, they are not combing through your hair or looking at it when it's wet (which is usually when *everyone's* hair looks thinner). They probably can't see any obvious thinning because you've styled your hair to make it look its best. So try and enjoy yourself!

"I constantly compare my hair loss to others."

A lot of my patients with hair loss say that they continually look at everyone else's hair, especially when traveling by bus or train. When they see someone with more hair than them, they get jealous; when they see someone with less hair than them, they get frightened.

I tell them that just because someone else has very thin hair, even in their family, it doesn't mean that their hair will continue thinning. There may be other factors contributing to that person's hair loss that have no bearing on his or her condition.

In addition, there will always be other people who we perceive as better looking or more intelligent than ourselves. Concerning yourself about a person's "better" hair takes away from the fact that you are doing everything possible to help your condition and so, hopefully, to improve your hair quantity.

To be preoccupied with other people's hair creates stress and anxiety, which can lead to more problems.

"I constantly worry about my hair loss."

Some people worry about their hair loss from the moment they wake up to the moment they fall asleep. Their day revolves around the amount of hair they lose in the morning. If they only lose a few hairs, then it means that the day is wonderful (even if it's raining); if the hair loss is high, the day is terrible (even if it's sunny).

It's difficult not to worry, but as long as you are treating the problem and have friends, family members, and/or doctors who are supportive, some of your anxiety should be alleviated.

"I go out less because I can't style my hair like I want to."

One of my patients wouldn't watch his son play football because he was worried that when the wind blew, everyone could see his thinning hair. He didn't want to wear a hat because he thought that it caused more hair loss.

Hats do not make the hair fall out even if they are tight. They may cause some breakage if you are too rough with putting them on and taking them off (especially the finer, thinner hairs that are the product of genetic hair loss). So don't be afraid to wear a hat (or baseball cap); it will not cause more hair loss

For social events, make your hair presentable with gels and sprays. As long as you don't incorrectly use hair products or brush them out vigorously (they are water soluble, so it's best to wash them out in the shower), then use them as often you need to. The bottom line with your hair is that you want it to look its best when you leave the house. Do whatever you need to do (within reason) to attain a look that you are comfortable with.

"I feel that my hair loss is affecting my career."

People feel that losing their hair affects their chances at progressing in a career, but studies do not show this to be true. For instance, one study (see References and Further Reading) looked at the percentage of men in government with hair loss (because it was noticed that the percentage of men who were state governors and in U.S. Congress with hair loss was well below the national average). This study found no evidence that candidates with genetic hair loss were discriminated against during elections (in other words voters would vote for them irrespective of the amount of hair they had). It did find, however, that the under-representation was due to men with hair loss having a negative self-perception, which discouraged them from running for office.

I have also done studies on this topic for women in the workplace, and found similar results; there was no evidence that women with hair loss were discriminated against by their boss.

The summary of these studies is not to allow your hair loss to affect your self-esteem enough to think that you won't get promoted, because it doesn't make a difference to your boss. However, if you become less outgoing, it may affect your ability to do your job properly.

"My hair loss has limited my sexual activity."

Many people with hair loss have less self-esteem and, therefore, feel less attractive to others. They often date less, which reduces their sexual activity. This is true even with married couples and people in long-term relationships. Some partners (especially women) refuse to talk about their hair loss with their spouse or significant other for fear of being seen as less attractive or even ugly. They try to reduce the frequency of making love, as they are afraid that the closeness of sex will reveal that their hair is thinning. Also, a negative self-perception can lead them to feel less desirable and so not feel like having sex.

It is important to take as much care of your appearance as you did before losing hair. Although it may take you a little longer to get ready to go out, make the effort. Your hair looks thicker than you realize and others do not notice thinning hair as much as you think (see "I feel that other people are always staring at my hair." in this chapter). For those in a relationship, remember that your partner loves you for yourself, not for your hair.

"I've seen so many doctors about my hair loss and I'm still losing hair."

If you have seen many specialists and are still not getting the results you are looking for, ask yourself whether you've given their advice a chance. Did you follow their suggestions for at least three months? Sometimes there are no easy answers as to why you are losing hair, and there's no magic pill that will stop your hair loss overnight. Often hair loss is a chronic condition that needs to be treated over time. Moreover, there is no reliable cure or definite regrowth formula. Sometimes nothing can be done to regrow all your hair; however, the advice that you have been given may help stabilize or slow the continuance of the condition. Remember that left unchecked (without treatment), some hair-loss conditions will continue unabated. Even these "partial" successes are, in fact, helping your hair loss.

In addition, some treatments may help your hair look better cosmetically, the importance of which should not be underestimated.

"My physician/hair-loss specialist said some hurtful things about my hair loss."

Some of the things I've heard that have been said to people with hair loss have been extremely hurtful. You would think that a physician or specialist would have a better bedside manner or show some empathy, but unfortunately some practitioners don't grasp the fact that many people with hair loss are worried and upset.

I've heard of one hair-loss specialist who said to a woman, "You're halfway through your life, and you've lost half your hair ... that seems fair." You can imagine why she ran out of his office crying!

Another physician not only showed no sympathy for a man's hair loss but also doubled the insult when he said, "It's a shame you're so short. People wouldn't be able to see your hair loss if you were taller." As you might expect, the man felt like hitting the doctor!

Hair loss often contributes to a loss of self-esteem and increased anxiety and depression, so comments of this sort really aggravate people's concerns. What can you do if something like this is said to you? I suggest leaving the office immediately and complaining to the board through which the practitioner is licensed. Also, look for a professional who has been personally recommended to you by a friend. Lastly, try not to let it affect you. It is the specialist who has a problem.

IS YOUR HAIR LOSS AFFECTING YOUR QUALITY OF LIFE?

Is your hair loss affecting your everyday life and outlook? How can you find out and then keep track? This shortened questionnaire, based on the Kingsley Alopecia Profile© (a questionnaire used in many medical studies), will help document how much your hair loss is affecting your quality of life. It will also help monitor how you feel about your hair over time.

Quality Of Life Questionnaire

(Based on The Kingsley Alopecia Profile©; see References and Further Reading)

This questionnaire consists of fifteen statements that should take you only five minutes to complete and five minutes to analyze.

Choose the answer that best describes how you feel *today* about each of the statements by checking the relevant boxes. There are five answers for each statement to choose from, strongly agree, agree, neither agree nor disagree, disagree, and strongly disagree. The following are definitions of each choice:

- Strongly agree means that you feel the statement is relevant to you most of the time.
- Agree means that you feel the statement is relevant to you some of the time.
- Neither agree nor disagree means that you feel you have no opinion about the statement.
- Disagree means that you feel the statement is probably not relevant to you.
- Strongly disagree means that you feel the statement is not relevant to you at all.

Make sure that you fully complete the fifteen-statement questionnaire. You will find the scoring explanation at the end of the questionnaire.

1. I feel unattractive as a result of my hair loss.

strongly agree	agree	neither agree nor disagree	disagree	strongly disagree
[]	[]	[]	[]	[]

2. My hair loss has made me withdrawn.

strongly agree	agree	neither agree nor disagree	disagree	strongly disagree
[]	[]	[]	[]	[]

3. I feel that other people are aware of my hair loss.

strongly agree	agree	neither agree nor disagree	disagree	strongly disagree
[]	[]	[]	[]	[]

4. Unless a person is experiencing hair loss they could never truly understand what it's like.

strongly agree	agree	neither agree nor disagree	disagree	strongly disagree
[]	[]	[]	[]	[]

5. I constantly worry about my hair loss.

strongly agree	agree	neither agree nor disagree	disagree	strongly disagree
[]	[]	[]	[]	[]

6. My hair loss makes me depressed.

strongly agree	agree	neither agree nor disagree	disagree	strongly disagree
[]	[]	[]	[]	[]

☐

7. I go out less because of my hair loss.

strongly agree	agree	neither agree nor disagree	disagree	strongly disagree
[]	[]	[]	[]	[]

☐

8. I do not like people talking to me about my hair loss.

strongly agree	agree	neither agree nor disagree	disagree	strongly disagree
[]	[]	[]	[]	[]

☐

9. I compare my own hair loss with that of others.

strongly agree	agree	neither agree nor disagree	disagree	strongly disagree
[]	[]	[]	[]	[]

☐

10. Losing my hair has been the most disturbing event of my life.

strongly agree	agree	neither agree nor disagree	disagree	strongly disagree
[]	[]	[]	[]	[]

☐

11. I will only do activities that don't mess up my hair.

strongly agree	agree	neither agree nor disagree	disagree	strongly disagree
[]	[]	[]	[]	[]

☐

12. I feel my hair loss is affecting my career.

strongly agree	agree	neither agree nor disagree	disagree	strongly disagree
[]	[]	[]	[]	[]

☐

13. My hair loss makes me look older than I am.

strongly agree	agree	neither agree nor disagree	disagree	strongly disagree
[]	[]	[]	[]	[]

☐

14. I feel that my hair loss gives a poor impression to someone who meets me for the first time.

strongly agree	agree	neither agree nor disagree	disagree	strongly disagree
[]	[]	[]	[]	[]

☐

15. I am self-conscious about my hair loss.

strongly agree	agree	neither agree nor disagree	disagree	strongly disagree
[]	[]	[]	[]	[]

☐

To score the questionnaire, write in the Score boxes under each statement the following values:

-2 for strongly disagree
-1 for disagree
0 for neither agree nor disagree
+1 for agree
+2 for strongly agree

Add up the numbers, and put the sum in the *total* box with the *date* that you filled in the questionnaire. Use Table 3.1: Total for Quality of Life Questionnaire :

Table 3.1: Total for Quality of Life Questionnaire

Date	Total

The range of your total results can only be from -30 to +30. If you have a score outside this range, you have either entered the wrong number in each box or have added your total incorrectly. Review the pluses and minuses, as they can be a little confusing.

- If you have a score of -30 to -15, then your hair loss has probably had no impact on your daily life and you are most likely unconcerned about losing hair. If this is the case, I still suggest you consider seeing a hair-loss specialist to find out why you are losing hair. This will help prevent the condition worsening and check that your hair loss is not indicative of any health problems.
- If you have a score of -14 to 0, then your hair loss has probably had very little impact on your daily life and you are most likely only mildly concerned about losing hair. If this is the case, I suggest you see a hair-loss specialist to help find out why your hair is falling out.
- If you have a score of +1 to +10, then your hair loss has probably had a minor impact on your daily life and you are most likely moderately concerned about losing hair. In addition, your hair loss is beginning to affect your quality of life. If this is the case, I suggest you see a hair-loss specialist to find out why you are losing hair and to help you improve your quality of life.

- If you have a score of +11 to +20, then your hair loss has probably had a moderate impact on your overall daily life and you are most likely very concerned about losing hair. In addition, your hair loss is beginning to affect your quality of life in a significant way. If this is the case, I suggest you see a hair-loss specialist to find out why you are losing hair and to help improve your quality of life. You may also benefit from discussing your hair loss fears and concerns with a licensed psychologist or psychiatrist.
- If you have a score of +21 to +30, then your hair loss has probably had a severe impact on your daily life and you are most likely extremely concerned about losing hair. In addition, your hair loss is having a major effect on your quality of life. If this is the case, I suggest you not only see a hair-loss specialist to find out why you are losing hair but to also discuss your hair loss fears and concerns with a licensed psychologist or psychiatrist.

Retake this questionnaire every three to six months, especially after using a treatment, to see whether the impact your hair has on your life has changed.

I AM COPING BETTER WITH MY HAIR LOSS. WHAT SHOULD I DO NEXT?

You have now assessed whether you are losing excessive quantities of hair (Chapter 1). You have also evaluated the extent to which your hair loss is affecting your quality of life, you are beginning to cope with the problem, and you are trying to limit its effects on your everyday life (Chapter 2).

The next step is to find out what is causing your hair loss problem. Is it stress, genetics, or some deficiency in your diet? Who can advise you on your condition? Chapter 3 will discuss the most common causes of hair loss. It will also help you decide who to see for advice and what tests you should expect them to perform.

At the end of Chapter 3, you should have a good idea of why you have hair loss and be able to discuss these causes with your hair-loss specialist.

THREE

WHY YOU ARE LOSING HAIR

You feel that your hair is thinning and/or falling out. Now what should you do? Well, the first step is to find out *why* your hair is falling out. This will help point you in the right direction for choosing the treatments that are best for you. Therefore, make an appointment to see a hair-loss specialist such as a dermatologist or a qualified trichologist.

WHAT YOU SHOULD LOOK FOR IN A HAIR-LOSS SPECIALIST.

When searching for a hair-loss specialist, ask questions. Many people are afraid to ask the practitioner's office staff questions, for fear of sounding ignorant or being difficult. However, if you're worried about losing your hair, then you want to see someone who knows what he or she is talking about.

When you call an office, before making an appointment make sure that the replies to your questions make sense and that the person on the other end of the phone is helpful. Rightly or wrongly, if the secretary or receptionist is uncooperative, then it may indicate that the office in general (including the hair-loss specialist) could be unsupportive. Let's face it. If you need to call the office in the future about making further appointments or refilling prescriptions, the last thing you want to deal with is an unfriendly receptionist.

Dermatologists

Although dermatologists are physicians that treat the skin, hair, and nails, not all specialize in hair loss. Therefore, before making an appointment, make sure that the dermatologist is up-to-date with the most recent hair loss research and takes the psychological impact of hair loss as seriously as he or she should.

Hair loss can cause a lot of emotional stress, and a dermatologist may not be able to allot enough time during the appointment to discuss these emotional concerns. Find out whether a properly trained nurse or receptionist in the dermatologist's office has the role of helping you with emotional support.

Dermatologists are able to prescribe medicines that are not over the counter, such as Propecia for men or corticosteroids for conditions such as alopecia areata or psoriasis. Dermatologists can also do biopsies of the scalp, if the condition warrants that approach.

For more information about dermatology, visit the American Academy of Dermatology Website at: www.aad.org, the British Association of Dermatologists Website at www.bad.org.uk, or the Canadian Dermatology Association Website at www.dermatology.ca.

Trichologists

Many people call themselves trichologists (hair and scalp specialists), even if they haven't been properly certified or qualified through a prestigious trichology association, society, or institute. Therefore, I suggest you thoroughly check their credentials. Ask through which organization they got their certification, and then check with that institute's Website to make sure that they really are affiliated. Also, double-check their credentials if they claim to be "doctors," as only a handful of trichologists worldwide have PhDs (at the time of writing this book I am the *only* trichologist in North America with a PhD—please note that a valid PhD can only be gained through a reputable university).

Trichologists look at hair loss problems in a holistic way. They are trained in the life sciences and they evaluate clients on the basis of personal history, lifestyle, genetic factors, and environmental conditions. With this information, a trichologist can suggest individualized treatments, give nutritional advice, and recommend lifestyle changes to improve the health and appearance of the hair and scalp.

If your hair loss is causing you stress or affecting your quality of life, a competent trichologist should be able to genuinely empathize with you. He or she should also spend time advising you on how best to cope with your condition as part of the treatment regimen.

Like other para-medical (non-physician) health specialists such as nutritionists, a competent trichologist should work closely with your medical doctor to find out whether any medical problems are associated with your hair loss, such as thyroid disease or anemia. Your physician should be willing to work with your trichologist in respect to taking and analyzing blood tests that your trichologist may suggest.

For more information about trichology, visit the Institute of Trichologists Website at www.trichologists.org.uk, the International Association of

Trichologists Website at www.trichology.edu.au, or The Trichological Society Website at www. hairscientists.org.

WHAT YOU SHOULD EXPECT FROM YOUR HAIRLOSS SPECIALIST.

As there could be *many* things causing your hair loss, it is important that the specialist you see spends time with you (I usually see a patient for thirty to sixty minutes during the initial evaluation). The specialist should look at your hair and scalp, take a full medical/lifestyle history, suggest blood tests, help you cope with your condition, and discuss all of your treatment options. Sometimes, the specialist needs to eliminate one factor before moving on to the next. Remember, many different factors may cause your hair to fall out. It is important to find each one so that any treatment you receive will be more effective.

The Specialist Should Look at Your Hair.

This may sound obvious, but you would be surprised by how many of my patients have said that a specialist they had seen either didn't look at their hair at all or only quickly glanced at it. The specialist should look at both your hair and scalp to see the distribution of your hair thinning, which can often indicate why it is falling out. By comparing the partings at different positions—for instance, the crown area, front area, sides, and back—differences in hair quantity can be seen and the amount of thinning can be determined. The distribution of hair would indicate the presence of a genetic condition, traction hair loss (also known as hair breakage), amongst other conditions (the most common types of hair loss are discussed in the Appendix). The specialist should also do a pull test in different areas of your scalp to see how much hair is coming out (the pull test is discussed in more depth later in this chapter).

I often look at the type of hairs growing from the scalp using a microscope program connected to my computer. With this I can see how many of the hairs have become finer in diameter, which often helps me in my assessment. I also look for the quantity of regrowth and whether the hairs are tapered at the tip or flat ended. The former would indicate a new hair, the latter a cut or broken hair. A lot of broken hair may indicate that cosmetic factors contributed to the hair loss.

Also, the specialist may look at the hair under a regular microscope (usually a trichologist will do this) or take a biopsy of the scalp (only a physician is able to do this).

The Specialist Should Look at Your Scalp.

It is also important for the specialist to look at the scalp to see whether there is any flaking, itching, redness, acne -like breakouts, or other lesions. Although a lot of scalp conditions don't cause hair loss and are just cosmetically annoying, some can increase hair shedding or indicate what is causing the hair loss problem.

You should be asked whether you have any periodic scalp tenderness (called *trichodynia*). The scalp can be sensitive for many reasons, so it is important for the specialist to ascertain the possible cause.

If you are in doubt about any scalp condition, or if your scalp feels constantly tender for any length of time (such as more than a few days), I suggest you see a specialist.

The Specialist Should Show Empathy

The specialist should be concerned about your condition. You're worried about losing hair, and this can often lead to anxiety and depression (see Chapter 2). The last thing you need is to be told that "It's all in your head" or "You've still got plenty of hair, so don't worry". The amount of hair that you've lost is relative to you, not other patients of the specialist. Also, you want to make sure that every possibility is explored in finding why you are losing your hair. Because hair loss is not a life-threatening illness, many physicians are indifferent. Yet hair loss often affects your quality of life, so it's important that your concerns are taken seriously.

The Specialist Should Sometimes Suggest Blood Tests

Blood tests can be an important diagnostic tool for hair loss. If I feel that tests are necessary, I send my patients to their primary care physician with a list of the ones I think are necessary. I usually suggest that their physician do a full thyroid screen, including thyroid -stimulating hormone, T4 (thyroxine) and T3 (triiodothyronine), as well as a blood profile that includes a CBC (complete blood count), iron, ferritin (iron stores), transferrin, TIBC (total iron-binding capacity), vitamin B12, ESR (erythrocyte sedimentation rate), and serum folic acid. Some of these tests should help the physician look for a condition of anemia or iron deficiency, a cause of hair loss for women that can also occur with men who are vegetarian. Depending on the medical/ lifestyle history, other tests that may be prudent for their physician to carry out are ANA (anti-nuclear antibodies) to test for lupus or other autoimmune conditions, and a hormone profile (other than thyroid) to see whether there are adrenal or pituitary problems.

For men, a testosterone profile including free testosterone, % free testosterone, total testosterone, DHT (dihydrotestosterone), DHEAS (dehydroepiandrosterone sulfate), and SHBG (sex hormone binding globulin) may be required.

For women who notice more facial or body hair or erratic menstrual cycles, a similar testosterone profile may be necessary, plus some other hormone tests such as 17-alpha-hydroxyprogesterone, estradiol, prolactin, LH (luteinising hormone), and FSH (follicular stimulating hormone).

The Specialist Should Assess Your Hair Loss

There are many different techniques that can be used to assess what type of hair loss condition you have. They can be used individually or in combination.

Microscopic Hair Root Analysis

When undertaken by a properly trained professional, a microscopic hair root analysis can be a useful method for helping find certain hair-loss conditions such as alopecia areata, traction alopecia, and cicatricial alopecia (see Appendix).

However, in the hands of untrained professionals, this method can cause confusion particularly when analyzing the anagen (growing) and telogen (resting) phases of the hair cycle (see the Appendix).

For example, some of my patients have told me that they had a hair analysis that looked at the root of their hair to see whether it was in the growing or resting phase. They were told that if the shape of the root looked like the bulb of a plant, then it was a healthy, growing hair; however, if the root was irregularly shaped, the hair was weak and in its resting phase. After the analysis, they were told that a majority of the hairs were in the resting (telogen) phase of the cycle because of their distorted shape, so there was a hair growth problem present.

Unfortunately, what they were told was incorrect. In fact, the opposite is true! A growing (anagen) root is a very pliable, soft tissue, because it contains living cells for the first two millimeters or so (one-tenth of an inch) from the papilla (the part of the follicle from where it grows). When the hair is pulled out, this tissue at the root stretches and then breaks away from the papilla, like a rubber band. As the tissue hardens in the air and is viewed under the microscope or magnifying lens, it has an irregular look. Also, it is often pigmented and is surrounded by a *translucent* (see-through) root sheath. A resting (telogen) root, on the other hand, has already hardened in the hair follicle and its bulb shape doesn't change when pulled out. When viewed under a microscope, the area where the shaft meets the root appears regularly shaped and has a small bulb shape, often without pigment or with less pigment than the rest of the hair shaft. This is what looks like a "plant bulb".

Scalp Biopsy

A dermatologist will often use this method to help with a diagnosis, particularly if he or she suspects that an inflammatory condition is causing the hair loss. The skin/follicle sample is sent to a laboratory that microscopically examines the sample and assesses possible causes for the condition. The lab can look for inflammation, white blood cell count, structural irregularities, and so on. This method is sometimes used in combination with a hair root analysis.

The disadvantage of a scalp biopsy is that once the follicles are removed, the area becomes scarred and hair cannot grow from it. Usually, however, only a very small incision is taken and so cannot be seen.

Microscopic Hair Shaft Analysis

The difference between hair shaft analysis and hair root analysis is that in the former, the mineral content of the hair is assessed instead of the shape of the root. This form of testing can be inaccurate. Therefore, check that the lab has no affiliation with a vitamin company because often deficiencies are found that are meaningless to hair loss yet are used to sell you supplements to help cure it. This method of testing for deficiencies should be done in combination with blood tests.

Trichogram

A trichogram is usually carried out in two ways: taking a picture of an area of the scalp and counting the hairs on a computer (*phototrichogram)* or plucking hairs from a measured area and assessing them under a microscope (*unit area trichogram).*

Trichograms can count the hairs to see whether the number is in the normal range per scalp area, and they can also help ascertain what percentage of hairs have become finer—often a diagnostic tool for genetic hair loss (if a large percentage of hairs are shorter than thirty millimeters in length and/or finer than forty microns in diameter, they are termed as nonmeaningful hairs, or hairs that do not add to the cosmetic appearance of the hair). The trichogram can also assess whether the percentage of hair in the growing and resting phases is abnormal (this latter assessment is more accurately done with the unit area technique).

With the unit area trichogram, hair is plucked (similar to having your eyebrows plucked) from an area of the scalp. This can cause discomfort both physically (it can be painful if not done correctly) and mentally (you're looking to stop your hair fall, not have it plucked out!). The phototrichogram can be just as effective as the unit area trichogram but with minimal discomfort (see References and Further Reading). Also, the unit area trichogram is best used for assessing the effectiveness of treatment regimens over time rather than purely for diagnosis, which, in the case of genetic hair loss, can be assessed by more conventional, cheaper, and less invasive means (such as the specialist visually assessing hair distribution).

Hair Pull Test

Most specialists will assess the rate of your hair loss by pulling at the hair in different places on your head. The best way for them to do this is to pinch a small sample of hair between the thumb and forefinger and pull firmly. The amount of hair that comes out will indicate the severity of the hair loss (the Hair Pull Test is also discussed in Chapter 5 under the "Pull Technique" heading).

More hair loss in different areas of the scalp might indicate some of the causes of the condition. For instance, whether it is falling locally (in one area) or in a diffuse manner (all over) may indicate the type of hair-loss condition you have.

Whilst having the hair pull test, you should be asked when your hair was last washed. This will give a more accurate assessment; as the longer ago your hair was washed, the more hair that would be expected to come out (the reason for this is discussed in greater depth in Chapter 1).

QUESTIONS YOU SHOULD BE ASKED DURING YOUR INITIAL CONSULTATION

Medical and Lifestyle History

During the initial evaluation the specialist should ask you a series of questions to help him or her find out what could be causing the loss or thinning. Not all questions you are asked will seem relevant, though often the answer is needed to rule out certain things. I tell my patients that sometimes finding the causes of hair loss is like detective work; we need to eliminate some "innocent" influences so that we can look for the "guilty" factors.

Before asking specific questions based on your health and lifestyle, I ask the following general questions.

How Long Have You Been Losing Hair?

Often the trigger of hair loss occurs between four and sixteen weeks (an average of three months) previous to you seeing the hair falling out. For instance, if you see a hair falling out in the wash in, say, June, that hair probably stopped growing in March. This is because when the hair goes into the resting (telogen) phase, it usually takes this amount of time for it to move into the falling out (exogen) stage.

Has the Hair Loss Been Continuous?

The answer to this question will indicate whether the cause has been continuously, or only periodically, affecting the hair cycle. Continuous influences could be genetic or a chronic general health condition. Periodic loss could indicate a dietary or stress influence.

When Did You Wash Your Hair Last?

This would indicate to me how much I should expect to see during the hair pull test. As discussed in Chapter 1, the frequency of washing corresponds to the amount of hair accumulation you should expect.

The 7 Hs of Hair Loss

I base the health and lifestyle questions that I ask my patients on my 7**H**s: the "7**H**s of Hair Loss©". This simple reference (all beginning with the letter "**H**" for Hair) is not exhaustive, but it covers many of the common causes of hair loss for both men and women. As you will see, some of the 7**H**s overlap, and so one question can help answer more than one of the 7**H**s. Also, your hair loss is often caused by more than one of the 7**H**s, so I always ask questions about each one to be thorough. As I will discuss later, some of the 7**H**s can cause permanent hair loss, while others cause only temporary hair loss.

Although I ask questions about all of the 7**H**s, some hair-loss specialists may not feel it necessary to do so. For instance, if you have genetic hair loss, many specialists will not bother to ask about your diet or stress levels as, in their minds, the cause is cut and dried. However, it should be noted that some nongenetic factors might accelerate a genetic condition. In genetic hair loss (see the Appendix), the hair fiber thins or becomes finer due, in part, to the hair follicle shrinking over time. Some researchers believe that the follicle becomes smaller only during the telogen (resting) phase, rather than during the anagen (growing) phase of the hair cycle. Therefore, if something besides genetics is causing your hair to fall out prematurely, and so causing the hair to enter the resting phase earlier than normal, it is logical that any genetic thinning may be accelerated. This is why I believe it is still important for a specialist to ask questions about other possible influences on the hair cycle.

H1. Heredity

This is the most common cause of hair loss in both men and women.

Hereditary or genetic influences on the hair follicle are talked about the most when an article or news feature mentions hair loss. But how important is the genetic link between you and your mother's hair or your father's hair or even your aunt's, uncle's, or grandparent's hair? Most experts would agree that genes passed down to you from your parents play a big role in hair loss but are not, in and of themselves, guaranteed to make you lose your hair.

Obviously, if most of the people in your family—whether on your mother's or father's side—are losing hair, then you have an increased chance of also losing hair. However, I know of many instances where both the mother and father have hair loss and the adult son and daughter do not. It can also work the other way. I see many patients complaining of losing their hair in a genetic like pattern, yet no one in their family on either side is bald or even thinning. In fact, in my experience, about 15 percent of people exhibiting genetic hair loss don't have *any* known family members with the condition (some reports have indicated that it could be as high as 20 percent—see References and Further Reading).

Besides the uncertainty of which hair-loss genes you are going to receive from your family, the type of hair loss is also important when discussing hereditary influences on the hair. Male pattern alopecia and female pattern hair loss are the most common hair-loss conditions connected with heredity factors, so there is definitely a very strong link between these type of hair-loss conditions and genetic influences. However, there is also a link, albeit much weaker, between heredity influences and, say, alopecia areata or traction alopecia.

How do you know whether you are going to have thinning hair like a certain member of your family or a full head of hair like another family member? It is impossible to say for sure whom you'll end up resembling in terms of the amount of your hair, as it depends on many factors. As a general guide, the more close family members that have a particular type of hair loss, the higher your chance of also developing the condition. Moreover, your hair loss will tend to look similar to a person in your family with similar hair characteristics to yourself. Characteristics to look for are the color of the hair, the hair type (for instance, coarse or fine), the hair texture (dry and curly or limp and straight), and the distribution of the hair on the scalp (thick or thin).

The subject of what side of a family (either the mother's or father's) will most likely pass its hair-loss genes on to the children is still controversial. For many years, it was thought that, irrespective of the sex of the child, the main hair-loss genes came from the mother's side of the family. However, some recent studies have indicated that these genes can come from either side of the family equally. Other studies indicate, more specifically, that a young man will more likely follow the hair pattern of his father's side of the family and a young woman will more likely follow the hair pattern of her mother's side (see References and Further Reading). Remember that these are generalizations and, as with most genetic conditions, no definite conclusions can be drawn.

In addition, genetic hair loss could be caused by more than one gene (called *polygenic*), so you may find that *both* sides of your family influence your hair loss. Your hair color and texture could also be a combination of your maternal and paternal hair types.

With all these scenarios it's easy to see why genetic hair loss can be so complicated to ascertain. This is why it's necessary for the specialist to ask you about both sides of your family. Therefore, I ask about your mother and father's hair, both sets of grandparents, and even your aunts' and uncles' hair. All can be relevant when assessing genetic hair loss.

Men's Genetic Hair Loss

Men's genetic hair loss is caused, in the main, by a sensitivity of the hair follicle to the male hormone dihydrotestosterone (DHT). The DHT (which is converted from the hormone, testosterone) causes the growing phase of the hair cycle to become shorter and, consequently, the resting phase to become longer. There is also a reduction in the size of the affected follicles causing the hair to become increasingly shorter and finer.

Most men see male pattern hair loss before they are thirty, although it can develop in later years. The hair usually begins to recede at the temples of your hairline or in the crown area. In advanced stages (which not all genetic hair-loss conditions reach), the whole top of the head, including the front and crown areas, thins out (see the Appendix for an in-depth discussion of genetic hair loss).

Women's Genetic Hair Loss

Female pattern hair loss, as with male pattern alopecia, is often triggered by the hair follicle's genetic sensitivity to normal levels of male hormones (such as DHT). The DHT produces premature hair loss and a gradual thinning of some of the hair fiber s. This miniaturization of the hair fiber s is less uniform than men and so, in the main; women do not exhibit a male pattern thinning.

In addition to DHT, some research has suggested that a reduction in the activity, or amount, of an enzyme called aromatase in the hair follicle (which converts male hormones to female hormones) may also contribute to female pattern hair loss (see References and Further Reading). This could account for the difference in clinical appearance between male pattern alopecia and female pattern hair loss.

Female pattern hair loss is typically diffuse (evenly spread over the scalp). Often a band of slightly denser hair is retained along the frontal hairline. Also, women can exhibit a "Christmas-tree" pattern, a normal area of hair at the front of their scalp that gradually thins out as you look further back near their crown (see References and Further Reading).

Women can be affected by genetic hair loss at any age after puberty. However, if there is no underlying hormonal problem, hair loss usually begins around menopause because of changes in the female-to-male hormone ratio (see the Appendix for an in-depth discussion of genetic hair loss). Although significantly fewer women, percentage-wise, have genetic hair loss when compared to men, many researchers believe that there are still a large number of women who suffer from this condition (see References and Further Reading).

Other Hair Loss Conditions

Many of my patients with male or female pattern hair loss also have other types of hair-loss conditions, such as, telogen effluvium (hair shedding) and traction alopecia (hair breakage). As these other hair-loss types can sometimes look clinically similar to genetic hair loss or, as some specialists believe, they can actually accelerate the genetic hair-loss condition, they often make the hair loss look worse (see References and Further Reading). Therefore, it is important to explore all underlying reasons for your hair loss.

H2. Health

I often use the following saying when discussing the effects of general health on the hair cycle : "The health of your hair is a barometer of your overall health."

So many health factors can influence your hair cycle. During your evaluation, besides asking about your general health, the hair-loss specialist should also ask you whether you have a family or personal history of a thyroid condition or anemia, two of the most common causes of hair loss next to genetics. Also, you should be asked whether you have had any recent blood tests taken within six to nine months (if you have, take a copy on your initial visit or send a copy at a later date). This will help the specialist know what other tests to suggest (see "The Specialist Should Sometimes Suggest Blood Tests" earlier in this chapter).

As mentioned earlier in this chapter, I try to work closely with my patients' family physicians by having them perform the required testing.

Other important health influences on your hair cycle include any recent surgery near the time the hair loss started; as anesthesia can disturb the hair cycle, as can the reason why you had the surgery in the first place. A high fever can also be a factor. A temperature greater than 101 degrees Fahrenheit (40 degree Celsius) can cause the hair to shed.

Obviously, numerous other general health factors can be important. For example, lupus (an autoimmune disease), digestive problems, and infections may be relevant to your condition. The most important health influences are often the ones that occurred approximately four to sixteen weeks before you noticed your hair falling out.

To try to determine the possible health factors that could have caused your hair loss, write down any illnesses that you have had, either chronic (over a period of time) or short term. Make a note of when the illnesses started, how long they lasted, and any medications that you took (or are taking) for them. Then work forward three months or so to see whether that was when your hair loss began. If you noticed that your hair began to fall out approximately three months after an illness, that illness might be one of the causes of your hair loss.

H3. Hunger (Nutrition)

Recent published research (see References and Further Reading) has shown that your hair needs a plentiful supply of protein, energy-producing molecules (glucose), and certain vitamins and minerals for optimal growth to occur. As the hair follicle is a nonessential tissue and, therefore, one of the last tissues to receive nutritious substances (or the first to have them reduced), any long-term deficiencies may lead to premature hair loss. Also, hair is one of the fastest-growing tissues in the body (it grows about a half inch each month), so any long-term reduction in certain nutrients to the hair follicle may disturb the hair cycle. Any nutritional disturbance to the hair follicle can cause the growing (anagen) phase of the hair cycle to become shorter, leading to an increase in shedding, and cause the resting (telogen) phase to become longer, slowing regrowth.

Protein deficiency can be a frequent cause for hair loss because insufficient levels of protein will reduce an essential raw material for hair growth. Protein helps the body build the hair fibers, which consist of 80 to 95 percent protein.

This is especially relevant for vegetarians or people who eat infrequently during the day (see the Appendix under "Hair Structure").

Eating infrequently or missing meals can adversely affect your hair cycle. If you do this over time, the amount of energy available at your hair growth site may be deficient, causing the hair to fall out prematurely.

The most common nutritionally related hair loss occurs while dieting. Severe weight loss due to dieting can often cause a temporary increase in hair shedding due to metabolic changes in the body. It has been reported that losing an excess of fifteen pounds of weight in a month can be a trigger for hair loss (see References and Further Reading). The loss usually begins two to four months after the onset of the diet; however, the hair tends to regrow to its original fullness another two to six months after the weight has been stabilized.

Anemia or iron deficiency is a common cause of hair loss, particularly for menstruating women and for men and women who are vegetarians. A blood test showing a low ferritin (iron storage) result may indicate that this could be a factor in causing your hair loss. Some researchers have suggested that not only can low iron stores cause hair loss, but they can also reduce the effectiveness of any hair-loss treatments (see References and Further Reading). If you think that your ferritin level may be low, speak to your physician.

The good news is that, usually, any short term deficiencies cause only temporary hair loss. Once corrected, hair will regrow normally. However, long-term shortages can occasionally lead to permanent hair loss as well as the acceleration of genetic hair loss, if present.

Heavy metals such as mercury, found in contaminated fish, can cause hair loss. Again, a blood test would generally help find out whether this is relevant to your condition.

H4. Hassle (Stress)

Stress can affect your hair cycle, and losing your hair can cause a lot of stress! However, which one triggers the other? Did the stress of meeting that deadline last month cause you to lose some hair, or was it the hair you noticed on your pillow last week that triggered the stress?

The exact role of stress as it relates to different types of hair loss is difficult to assess accurately. Under most circumstances, as with many other hair-loss causes, increased hair shedding occurs between four and sixteen weeks after the trigger has occurred. Yet most people attribute an increase in hair shedding to what happened yesterday or last week, not a couple of months ago. If your stress levels are normal at the time you see your hair thinning, you are unlikely to associate your problem with a stressful situation that occurred, say, three months before. Although it is difficult to pinpoint a specific stress episode as the cause of hair loss, there is evidence (see References and Further Reading) that acute and chronic stress may precipitate hair-loss conditions, such as genetic hair loss, telogen effluvium (hair shedding), and alopecia areata (patchy hair loss—see the Appendix).

When asked, most people say they are under a "normal" amount of stress, so it can be difficult to assess whether this is affecting the hair. To help assess people's stress levels, I usually ask them to rate their stress levels one to three months before they started noticing their hair fall on a scale of 1 to 10 with 10 being the most stress. If the hair loss occurred periodically over a long span of time, then I would ask if and when there had been greater stressful episodes, and then try to correlate these with the hair loss.

In addition to stress causing hair loss, hair loss undoubtably causes stress for the sufferer. It affects one's self esteem and quality of life, which in turn can cause more hair loss. I have discussed this further in Chapter 2.

H5. Healing (Medications)

Taking certain medicines can cause hair loss in some people while the same medicine may not cause hair loss in others. Stopping a certain medicine can also cause hair loss in some, but not in others. In addition, certain medications can cause hair fall the first time they are taken, but not subsequent times (once the body adjusts to the medicine, the hair loss stops), or they don't cause hair loss the first time but do subsequent times (possibly due to the medicine accumulating in your system).

Sound complicated?

It is difficult to categorically say that one particular medicine causes hair loss and another doesn't, as medicines can react differently in different people. For instance, a medicine for blood pressure caused hair loss in one of my patients (his hair starting falling out ten weeks after starting the medicine), but that same medicine did not cause hair loss in another male patient. Also, stopping the contraceptive pill in one female patient caused hair loss about six weeks later, whereas another patient stopped the pill and lost no hair because of it.

So what particular groups of medications have been reported to cause hair loss?

The most common ones are:

- **Chemotherapy medications.** These can cause temporary hair loss by stopping the hair growth almost immediately (called *anagen effluvium*). They can also produce changes in hair texture, hair type, and pigmentation

- **Antidepressants.** In particular, lithium-based medicines can temporarily disturb the hair cycle and cause hair loss.
- **Thyroid medicines.** Both an under-active (*hypothyroid*) and an over-active (*hyperthyroid*) condition can cause the hair to fall out, as can the initial use of a thyroid medicine. Often, when a person starts taking thyroid medicine, the physician will need to vary the dosage until the correct balance is found. Some people experience hair loss during this process, up until three to six months after the dosage has been stabilized.
- **Oral contraceptive pill.** Either stopping or starting the pill may cause hair cycle disturbances. Oral contraceptives can affect the hormone levels, which often control hair growth.
- **Other groups of medicines.** Other medicines that can cause hair loss include blood pressure medications (blood thinners and beta blockers); cholesterol medicines; medications for ulcers, gout, arthritis, and Parkinson's disease; and anticonvulsants (for epilepsy).
- **Vitamins and supplements.** Some of these can cause hair loss such as taking too much vitamin A (in excess of 25,000 IU per day) and taking excessive quantities of 'natural' testosterone boosters.

I'm frequently asked the following questions about the instructions on or in the package of a particular medication.

"If the medication says 'may cause hair loss' on the package, will it definitely cause hair loss?"

Just because the small print on the package says a medication *may* cause hair loss doesn't mean that it will for you. As mentioned earlier in this section, people respond differently to different medicines. Also, the hair loss may be caused by the disease or condition for which you are taking the medication in the first place.

I suggest discussing the side effects of any medicine with your doctor or pharmacist. You can then decide whether to take another medicine or continue with the one you are using. Obviously, if you need to take a certain medication for your general health, then any potential effects on your hair should be secondary. If changing your medication, give it three to six months to see whether your hair loss improves. You may find that it causes only a temporary fall and that once your system becomes used to it, the hair loss declines.

"If a medicine doesn't mention hair loss as a possible side effect, does it mean that it will not cause hair loss?"

As mentioned before, some medicines will affect people's hair in different ways. Even if hair loss is not one of the listed side effects, it may still be causing or contributing to your hair loss.

"If a medicine mentions that it causes hair loss, is it permanent?"

Usually, once the medicine is stopped the hair should cease falling out and regrow normally within six months or so. If you've taken the medication for many years, it is possible for the hair regrowth potential to be diminished.

H6. Hormones

Hormones control hair growth to a large extent. In H1. Hereditary, I explained the importance of the male hormones testosterone and dihydrotestosterone (DHT) on the hair cycle. In H2. Health and H5. Healing, I discussed that thyroid hormones can contribute to hair loss conditions. Many other hormonal irregularities can affect the hair cycle. Often these produce other symptoms that can indicate their presence, although even if there is an absence of any other symptoms, it does not rule out that a hormonal factor is present.

For Men

- **Anabolic steroids.** Men who are taking steroids to build muscle for weight training to bulk up often see more hair loss, particularly if they have a genetic propensity. This is often associated with increased acne, especially on the back. Some supplements that help in muscle development may also contribute to genetic hair loss.

For Women

For women, hormonal influences on their hair can be indicated by the presence of any of the following symptoms and conditions:

- **Irregular menstrual cycles.** If your periods are heavier or lighter or become erratic (such as, missing periods or getting too many), then you should undergo a hormonal check-up to assess whether there is an imbalance that may also be affecting your hair cycle.
- **Polycystic ovarian syndrome.** Many women with ovarian cysts also have hair loss. Sometimes a few chin hairs and ovulation discomfort can be present with the hair loss. Glucose intolerance and obesity can also be symptoms. Usually a sonogram of the ovaries is needed to confirm a diagnosis.
- **Oral contraceptive pill.** If you have recently started or stopped the oral contraceptive pill or changed brands, you may experience some

hair fall between six and sixteen weeks later. If stopping the pill, the hair loss is usually temporary. However, if you were taking the pill for medicinal purposes, such as correcting a hormonal imbalance, then stopping it may lead to more permanent loss. If starting or changing the pill, you could see some temporary hair loss. Although some pills do make hair loss worse, it is important to check with your physician or pharmacist regarding any potential side effects.

- **Post-partum (after giving birth).** There is often hair loss three to six months after having a baby. One explanatory theory is that many women become iron deficient during pregnancy. Another theory is that the hormone progesterone increases during pregnancy keeping the hair growing for longer—hence your hair often looks better during the pregnancy—and then the progesterone levels drop, causing the hair that should have fallen out during the previous nine months to do so all at once (see Reference and Further Reading). I suggest that my patients take a picture of their hair when they find out that they are pregnant and compare that hair with what their hair will look like after their post-partum hair loss, rather than with the way their hair was when they gave birth.
- **Menopause.** Women who are menopausal or perimenopausal (shortly before menopause) often experience hair loss from hormonal changes such as reduced estrogen and progesterone levels. This can trigger a genetic hair-loss condition or sometimes telogen effluvium (hair shedding).

For Men and Women

- **More body hair (hirsutism).** More hair on a woman's face, chest or abdomen may indicate a hormonal irregularity and cause the physician to run a hormonal profile. With men, more chest hair or stronger beard growth may be associated with hair loss on the scalp; the male hormone DHT causes the paradox of hair loss from the scalp but hair growth on the body.
- **Acne and excessive oiliness.** Often an increase in acne and facial or scalp oiliness can be indicative of more active hormones in the skin. This can be a sign of male hormone activity in both men and women.

H7. Hairdressing

Although not technically hair loss from the scalp, losing hair through breakage can cause thinning and slow growth. Breakage can occur due to chemical over-processing and/or incorrect styling, drying, or brushing techniques (see the H7. Hairdressing section in Chapter 4 and the in-depth discussion of hair breakage in the Appendix).

Using a dryer that is too hot can cause the hair to burn, often so much so that you can smell it burning as you dry. In addition, too hot of a dryer can boil the water in the hair shaft and cause "bubble hair," where the hair strand is weakened as bubbles form in the hair shaft. It's best to keep the dryer at arm's length and in constant motion. A hot dryer can also burn the scalp, especially if the hair is thinning. Remember this saying, "If it hurts, it harms."

Vigorous brushing can also cause the hair to break. Comb first to detangle the hair by moving the comb through the ends first and then gradually up the shaft, combing in downward strokes. Then use a brush for styling, if needed. Finer hairs tend to be more prone to breakage than coarser hairs.

WHAT TO EXPECT AT THE END OF THE INITIAL ANALYSIS

You should expect one of two things. Either you have blood tests and return to the specialist's office for a follow-up appointment, or you are told there and then the causes for your hair loss problem. During both scenarios, the treatments needed to rectify the problems should be discussed.

I usually send my patients to their primary care physicians for blood work, as I feel that the more information that is available the better I am able to make recommendations.

During your follow-up appointment (or during your initial appointment if no further tests are necessary), you should expect the hair-loss specialist to discuss all the factors that could be causing your loss. As there could be more than one reason for losing your hair, you may be recommended to use more than one treatment regimen (see chapter 4).

WHAT YOUR HAIR SPECIALIST SHOULD EXPECT FROM YOU

- Arrive punctually to fill in any information that may be necessary.
- Write down any questions that you want to ask so that you don't forget anything. This also makes the time you have in the office more efficient.

- Write down medications and supplements that you may be taking so that you are ready to answer any questions about them.
- Have a time line of your condition, particularly of when it started and when it worsened (or improved) previously.
- Be succinct, as you probably have only a short time with the specialist.

Keep a Diary

Often, it can be difficult to assess exactly all the factors that are either causing or contributing to you hair loss. It is possible that you'll never know for sure all the factors, but there is a good chance that you'll find most of them. Sometimes I suggest that you keep a diary to record all the information that can affect your hair cycle. On each day, write what you ate, your stress levels from 1 to 10 (10 being high), any medicines you started or stopped, and for women, when you had your periods. After three months or so, I often find a pattern that could be influencing someone's hair cycle.

What Questions You Should Ask The Hair Loss Specialist

As I mentioned earlier, don't be frightened or intimidated to ask questions. If you are rushed out of the office or the specialist makes you feel uncomfortable when you question his or her treatments, then it may be a good idea to look for someone else to take care of your problem. You want to know what to expect, especially if you have to pay for the treatments.

Consider asking some of the following questions:

- What is causing my hair loss?
- How much hair should I see come back?
- How long will it take?
- How does the treatment work?
- How much will the treatment cost?

I KNOW WHY MY HAIR IS FALLING OUT, WHAT SHOULD I DO NEXT?

This chapter has helped you discover why your hair is falling out by discussing the main causes of hair loss. It has helped you decide whether you need to see a specialist and, if so, what type of tests to expect. It has advised you to ask questions so that you understand why your hair is falling out.

You may have found that there is more than one cause for your hair loss and that there may be more than one treatment necessary to help your condition. In Chapter 4, I have again used the 7Hs to discuss the different types of treatments that are available. Remember that if your hair loss is caused by more than one factor, it may be necessary to use a multiple-treatment approach to help the condition.

Chapter 4 will help you decide what treatments to choose to help your hair loss.

FOUR

TREATING YOUR HAIR LOSS

Once you find out why you are losing hair, you need to decide on what treatments to use, if any. If you look on the Internet, you'll find a host of different products promising to regrow your hair. Which one should you use? A lot of products are expensive versions of saw palmetto (an herb which may help to block the conversion of testosterone to DHT) or minoxidil, both of which you could probably get cheaper elsewhere.

It is important to realize that there is no *100 percent guarantee* with any treatment; as, at the writing of this book, no single treatment is available that will regrow *everyone's* hair. In fact, I would go so far as to say that if anyone offers a 100 percent guarantee, you should be extremely skeptical. This doesn't mean that there is no hope as there are many causes of hair loss. Depending on why your hair is falling out, there are many treatments that can improve your condition and regrow your hair. Sometimes you may need to change treatments or use more than one treatment to find the best combination for *you*. This is why it's important to find out what's causing your hair loss first.

TREAT THE CAUSES, NOT JUST THE SYMPTOMS

So what treatments should you use? The answer largely depends on what is causing your hair loss. Generic treatments, which you can purchase at many beauty salons and pharmacists, are formulated to help everyone with hair loss. They may temporarily help the symptoms of your hair loss, but if you don't identify the root of the problem, you will not see long-term improvement. Many treatments will help a proportion of people, but you want to use what will help *you* specifically. So, after you have ascertained why your hair is falling out, you want to use a treatment regimen that will help all these factors.

Often, therefore, a multifaceted treatment is necessary to get the best results. The more treatments that you use that are orientated to your problems, the better the chance of improvement.

FULL REGROWTH IS NOT THE ONLY MEASURE OF IMPROVEMENT

There are different levels of improvement. As the hair often deteriorates without treatment with some hair conditions, slowing down the loss or stabilizing it might actually be an improvement (compared to what would occur without treatments). With minoxidil, for instance, data has shown that even if you don't see regrowth, the percentage deterioration in hair quantity is often much less than if you hadn't used it at all (see References and Further Reading).

Of course, most people look for a slight improvement or, preferably, full regrowth from any treatment. There is always the possibility of curing your condition, however, depending on how long you have had the problem, you may have to look for an improvement that is between what your condition is *now* and what is was *before* you had the hair loss. Will this be enough to satisfy you? Time will tell. The longer you have had a hair loss-problem, the more difficult it may be for you to attain full regrowth.

GIVE TREATMENTS A CHANCE

In the previous chapter, I mentioned that hair loss often happens six to sixteen weeks after the trigger has occurred, so any treatment needs to be given the same length of time. If you are not willing to give a treatment regimen at least three months (after which time you should be seeing early results), I suggest you don't start using it in the first place; it's not fair on the treatment, or on your wallet.

DURATION OF TREATMENTS

How long should you keep using a treatment that seems to work? Many hair-loss conditions can be viewed as chronic (long term) conditions and just like any other chronic condition, treatment needs to be long term, especially with genetic hair loss. Therefore, you may need to use a treatment regimen consistently for it to continue working. For instance, if your hair loss is caused by dietary reasons, then you need to make sure that you keep following your corrected diet.

EVALUATING TREATMENT ADS

You've probably seen those wonderful photographs on the television or Internet of how much other people's hair has grown back from using certain treatments. If you look closely at some of these pictures, you may notice that some photographic tricks are being played.

For instance:

- **"Is the light exactly the same in both pictures"?**

You'll find that an overexposed picture will give the impression of less hair and that a slightly underexposed (darker picture) will give the impression of more hair. In addition, the hair may have been colored after treatment to give it a fuller appearance; where the roots are gray, the hair tends to look thinner.

- **"Is the angle at which both pictures were taken the same?"**

Changing the angle can make a big difference. Because you see more hair strands, a direct overhead picture of the scalp will look thinner than a picture taken at an angle. Like a forest, the trees will look thicker from ground level than they will from above—especially in the winter when there are fewer leaves.

- **"How much does the treatment cost?"**

Often, advertised treatments are more expensive than other available treatments. For instance, many ads that say a treatment helps reverse genetic hair loss just turn out to be expensive versions of minoxidil and saw palmetto (a herb).

TREATMENT CHOICES

I'm a firm believer that hair loss is best treated from both the inside and outside of the body. The best way to assess your treatment options is by using the "7**H**s of Hair Loss©" list.

H1. Heredity

As genetic hair loss is the most common cause of thinning, there are more products orientated to help this type of fall than for any other condition. Although none can guarantee regrowth, many have a better than 50 percent chance of working, so the odds are in your favor that you can achieve some improvement.

Even if a product will not help full regrowth, many can help slow the onset of the condition or provide some cosmetic aid.

In general, the younger people are when they begin to lose hair, the more they will lose; however, especially with men, they will still not necessarily lose all of it. It is also important to remember that not all hair loss is genetic, and even if your type is, it does not always mean that you are going to be bald. There are many different phases of genetic hair loss, from just a little thinning to almost complete loss. I see many people of all ages who, once they notice a little bit of hair thinning, feel that they are going to lose all of their hair. Obviously, some men do. However, most don't, and with women, total loss is extremely rare. Hair loss often stops at a phase well before total loss, even without any type of treatment.

Some of the most commonly used treatments for genetic hair loss include the following.

For Men

Propecia

Propecia (also known as finasteride and Proscar) is a pill that has also been FDA approved for men only. It was introduced in 1997 and requires a prescription from a dermatologist or other medical doctor. Propecia works by reducing the enzyme 5-alpha reductase (type II), which converts the male hormone testosterone to dihydrotestosterone (DHT). It is claimed that Propecia has over an 80% efficacy for male patients (see References and Further Reading).

During the clinical assessment of my patients, I have observed that when it is used in combination with minoxidil and/or laser therapy, the effectiveness of Propecia is enhanced. I use Propecia as part of an overall treatment strategy for my own hair loss (see the Preface).

It has been reported (see References and Further Reading) that 2 percent of men may experience side effects from Propecia, which are usually a reduction in sex drive and/or a reduction in sperm count. If you are affected in this way, stopping its use will help return both your libido and sperm count to normal.

A recent study (see References and Further Reading) indicated that Propecia may help some postmenopausal women but more research needs to be carried out before its effectiveness is confirmed.

Caution. Women who are or may potentially be pregnant must not use Propecia and should not handle crushed or broken Propecia tablets because the active ingredient may cause abnormalities of a male baby's sex organs. If a woman who is pregnant comes into contact with the active ingredient in Propecia, a doctor should be consulted.

Dutasteride

Also known as Avodart, dutasteride is a prescription medicine (usually prescribed for an enlarged prostate) that inhibits both the type I and type II 5-alpha reductase enzymes that convert testosterone to DHT (on the other hand, Propecia mainly inhibits type II). A recent study has shown dutasteride to be more effective in treating male pattern alopecia than finasteride (see References and Further Reading). At the time of writing this book, dutasteride has not been studied in women nor is it US FDA approved for the treatment of male pattern alopecia.

Saw Palmetto

The herb, *saw palmetto* (also called *Serenoa repens*), is often suggested instead of the prescription medicine finasteride (Propecia). There is some disagreement about its effectiveness for helping hair loss, as some studies have indicated that it may help reduce genetic hair loss while others suggest that it doesn't help (see References and Further Reading).

More studies need to be carried out, however, I feel that saw palmetto is a good, safe option for those who do not wish to use the prescription medicine, although it is not as effective as Propecia.

I have formulated a supplement, called *Hair Supplement Extra*, which contains saw palmetto as well as a combination of vitamins, minerals, and amino acids specifically for the hair (see http://www.hairandscalp.com/products-1loss.htm for more information).

For Women

Spironolactone

Also known as Aldactone, spironolactone appears capable of arresting the course of female pattern hair loss. A study that I co-authored in 1991 (see References and Further Reading) showed that hair loss stabilized for a group of women who took the medication orally for twelve months. When the spironolactone dosage was doubled for a further twelve months, increases in total and meaningful hair densities (cosmetically important hair) were reported.

The results of further studies have been mixed, and I suggest trying this medication only if there are other hyper-androgenic symptoms present besides the scalp hair loss, such as facial or body hair (*hirsutism*), acne, erratic periods, or excessive skin oiliness. A medical doctor must prescribe this medicine, and the dosage for helping hair loss should be between 100 and 200 milligrams per day.

For Men and Women

Minoxidil

Minoxidil was the first FDA-approved medicine for hair regrowth under the name Rogaine in 1988 (see References and Further Reading). It was approved for overthe-counter use (no prescription needed) in 1997. Usually the 5 percent solution is recommended for men and the 2 percent for women. It is applied topically (directly to the scalp) twice a day.

Many explanations have been given for how it works (see References and Further Reading). It has been suggested that the minoxidil may inhibit 5-alphareductase activity (the enzyme which converts testosterone to DHT), swell the hair shaft, dilate the blood vessels, darken the hair fiber, and open potassium channels (which may increase the cell's production of energy—ATP).

Many pharmacies and hair-loss experts have started producing their own generic minoxidil solutions, sometimes with additives for extra absorption. Some dermatologists have introduced stronger minoxidil solutions (more than a 5 percent solution). A number of them may work better, but others are just expensive versions of the original formulation.

Most minoxidil brands only claim to help the hair on the crown of the head, but many hair-loss specialists have also seen improvement when it has been used on the frontal hair.

If you decide to use minoxidil, you need to follow the instructions carefully and apply one milliliter twice daily to the thinning area. Be consistent with its use, or you are not giving it a fair chance. If you are unable (or forget) to use it twice a day, remember to use it a minimum of ten times a week, instead of the fourteen times that is prescribed (twice daily *x* seven days a week), or it will be ineffective. If you find that it's working, you need to continue its use or any improvement will fall out.

Using minoxidil can cause side effects. Women can sometimes get more facial hair (especially if they use the stronger 5 percent solution). Often this is caused by applying the solution too close to bedtime, which prevents it from drying properly before putting your head on the pillow. During the night the solution may spread from the pillow to your face, so causing this extra facial hair (if this is relevant to you, I suggest applying the solution a few hours before going to bed to allow it to dry). When applying minoxidil before blow-drying, you might get some on your face if you dry your hair with your head down (in this case, take extra care when drying your hair by keeping your hair away from your face until it is dry). If these steps do not work, and you decide to stop using the minoxidil, the facial hair growth will gradually subside.

Another side effect of minoxidil for both men and women is an itchy, flaky scalp. Often you can control this with special shampoos or topical treatments, but sometimes it causes such a problem that stopping its use is the only option.

An additional issue, especially for women, is that the solution can make the hair, flat or oily-looking. In this case, I suggest washing your hair more often to reduce this problem. Recently, a foam version of 5 percent (extra strength) Rogaine has been introduced which may help lessen these cosmetic problems.

Minoxidil is quite effective for genetic hair loss, so I often suggest that both my male and female patients use this treatment. I am using a 5 percent minoxidil solution as part of an overall treatment regimen for my own hair loss (see the Preface). I have found that combining minoxidil with other treatments enhances its effectiveness for genetic hair loss (see later in this chapter).

I have two strengths of mixoxidil that I use in my trichology centers: *Hair Therapy Extra*–containing 5% minoxidil and *Hair Therapy Regular*–containing 2% minoxidil (see http://www.hairandscalp.com/products-1loss.htm for more information).

Laser Light Therapy

Low-level laser light therapy is an over-the-counter treatment that has garnered attention in the past few years. It is a safe device that uses low-intensity phototherapy that is cool to the touch (rather than the hot, high-power lasers used in industry for cutting). In a published medical paper (see References and Further Reading), the HairMax LaserComb (one type of laser light therapy) was purported to encourage hair growth and improve the tensile strength of the hair fiber. It was discussed in this study that the improvement of the hair was possibly due to the therapy increasing microcirculation and also enhancing the hair papilla's ability (where the hair cells are formed) to produce cellular energy.

At first I was wary of the claims made about laser therapy. However, after trying the HairMax LaserComb machine on myself with good results and then using it on some of my patients, I was convinced that there was some benefit to this type of treatment.

In late 2002 the Canadian government approved the HairMax LaserComb as a medical device (Class 2) that helps stop hair loss and regrows hair. In January 2007, the United States FDA cleared the LaserComb as a device for the promotion of hair growth.

I often use this laser therapy device as one of the treatment options for both my male and female patients with good results. For treating my own genetic hair loss condition, I use the LaserComb as part of an overall treatment strategy (see the Preface). I have found that the effectiveness of each treatment is enhanced when the LaserComb is used with minoxidil and Propecia (for men only).

Anti-Androgen Therapy

Because the androgens (male hormones) testosterone and dihydrotestosterone (DHT) are important in triggering genetic hair loss, compounds with anti-androgenic activity (ones that reduce male hormones) can be very helpful in the treatment of the condition.

Cyproterone Acetate

One such anti-androgen, called Androcur, is a steroidal anti-androgen (also known as cyproterone acetate) that is available in Europe and Canada with a prescription, but not in the United States (see References and Further Reading). Androcur reduces free-circulating testosterone production and consequently reduces dihydrotestosterone (DHT). It has been shown to be effective in helping genetic hair-loss conditions (see References and Further Reading), although its main use is in treating prostate cancer.

One of the major problems in treating genetic hair loss with this type of anti-androgen therapy is the difficulty in predicting what effective dosage is required; the levels of circulating male hormones do not necessarily provide reliable information regarding the rate of change occurring in the scalp hair. Women can find cyproterone acetate in certain oral contraceptive pill s (which are also unavailable in the United States).

Progesterone

Another anti-androgen therapy that has been used with varying success in treating genetic hair loss is the female hormone, progesterone (see References and Further Reading). Used topically (in men and women) or systemically (only in women), progesterone may help reduce the amount of DHT that is converted from testosterone. Reports of the success of this treatment are limited.

Topical Niacin -Based Products

The effectiveness of topical niacin (vitamin B3) based products, such as nicotinic acid, may be beneficial for helping hair loss. A 2006 study (see References and Further Reading) concluded that there was a statistical improvement in the hair growth of women using a topical niacin solution when compared to a control group.

It is possible, therefore, that solutions containing topical niacin based ingredients can not only benefit hair loss but can also enhance the effectiveness of other treatments, such as laser therapy, minoxidil, and Propecia (men only).

I use a topical solution of nicotinic acid (called *Scalp Therapy*) as part of an overall treatment strategy for my own hair loss (see the Preface); and in some of the treatments that I use in my trichology centers (see http://www.hairandscalp.com/products-1loss.htm for more information).

H2. Health

Long-term general health factors that are affecting your hair can be more difficult to overcome because your hair cycle may be disturbed for the period of the illness. If you suffer from a long-term health problem that you think is causing hair loss, try and concentrate on as many of the other 7**H**s as possible to minimize the impact of the illness on your hair (see each section of the 7**H**s for more detailed advice). For instance, try to improve your overall lifestyle by eating healthy and exercising, as well as improving the look of your hair by washing or coloring it frequently.

Not all long-term illnesses cause hair loss. For the ones that do, some only affect the hair in the short term, after which the hair loss or thinning will stabilize and occasionally improve.

With short-term health problems such as a high fever, once the ailment has been cured and you have fully recovered, your hair should begin to improve a few weeks after you notice the start of the hair loss. Remember that the hair loss can begin four to sixteen weeks after the onset of the illness.

H3. Hunger (Nutrition)

There has been a lot of recent research into the effects of diet on hair loss (see References and Further Reading). As a result, you need to address many important issues when considering this "H" as a possible influence on your hair loss.

Hair is frequently termed as a non-essential tissue, meaning it is not important for the functioning of the body. Because of this, the hair is often the first thing that is nutritionally cut back on by the body or the last thing to receive its nutrition.

Hair is also one of the fastest-growing tissues in the body. If you pulled together all the hair that grows on your scalp in a month to form a single strand, the strand would be approximately 3/4 mile or 1 kilometer in length! Therefore, a lot of raw materials (such as protein) are needed to help your hair grow, in addition to an adequate supply of energy (such as simple carbohydrates).

Protein (Raw Materials for Hair Growth)

I suggest that to maintain an adequate amount of protein to help maximize your hair growth potential, you should eat at least 5 ounces (approximately 150 grams) of protein a day. You can eat protein in many forms, including meat, chicken, fish, beans, and tofu. Because your hair is made of 80 to 95 percent protein, this is an area of your diet that needs to be addressed.

Certain amino acids (substances that make proteins) are also important for our hair, especially l-lysine and l-cysteine. These can be taken as a supplement. I suggest taking 500 milligrams of l-lysine and 250 milligrams of l-cysteine per day.

Although I suggest protein in your diet, I do not advocate very high-protein, low-carbohydrate diets. I believe your hair needs a balance. With too little protein, your body may lack the raw materials to build your hair; with too little carbohydrates, your body may lack enough "fuel" to drive the machinery that produces your hair.

Carbohydrates (Glucose —Energy for Hair Growth)

Glucose, a simple carbohydrate or monosaccharide, is used by our cells to make energy (called ATP). The liver maintains a constant level of glucose in the blood and stores several hours' (approximately four to five hours) reserve in the form of glycogen. Therefore, you need to eat regularly (every four hours) to maintain adequate energy levels for your hair follicles. I usually suggest to my patients to either eat six small meals per day or to have three meals supplemented with small snacks in between each.

Glucose is a simple carbohydrate that can be derived from more complex carbohydrates such as fruits, vegetables, breads, and pasta.

Minerals and Vitamins

Normal hair growth also requires adequate amounts of minerals and vitamins in your diet. You should eat these in a balanced diet (see *Lifestyle Diet)* and, if necessary, take them in the form of supplements.

Iron deficiency is a major cause of hair loss in women, so if a woman is iron deficient or anemic, then taking iron could be helpful for her hair. To find out whether you are iron deficient or anemic, see your physician for a blood test.

I have formulated a supplement, called *Hair Supplement for Women,* which contains iron as well as a combination of other minerals, vitamins, and amino acids (see http://www.hairandscalp.com/products-1loss.htm for more information).

Also, an adequate amount of B complex vitamins —such as biotin (100 to 500 micrograms per day), vitamin B12 (25 to 200 micrograms per day), and folic acid (200 to 400 micrograms per day)—can help the hair. Biotin can be found in oatmeal, egg yolk, and soy; vitamin B12 in dairy, meat, and fish; and folic acid in beans, grains, vegetables, and fruit.

Other important minerals and vitamins for healthy hair functioning are: zinc (found in seafood and cereals), silica (found in potatoes, red and green peppers, and bean sprouts), magnesium (found in green vegetables and nuts), and essential fatty acids (such as omega fatty acids found in fish). You can take these individually or in a one-a-day supplement.

Beware of taking too much vitamin A (in excess of 25,000 IU per day). It can cause hair loss if taken in extremely high dosages.

Nourkrin

As well as recommending my nutritional supplements to patients, I often suggest that they also take a marine-protein based supplement called Nourkrin. Developed by scientists in Scandinavia, Nourkrin has been shown to help improve hair growth in clinical studies (see References and Further Reading). I use Nourkrin as part of my own treatment regimen (see the Preface) and have also seen it produce good results when used as part of my patients' treatment therapy.

Caution. Before taking any supplements, see a knowledgeable practitioner, physician, or healthcare provider.

Lifestyle Diet

I suggest that you follow a general lifestyle diet rather than continually dieting as rapid weight gain or loss can cause hair loss (see H3. Hunger in Chapter 3). This means that you should try and eat balanced meals every day, not just when you decide to go on a diet. Frequent (six) small meals or three meals supplemented with regular snacks are the best type of "lifestyle diets".

Consult with a registered dietician or your primary care physician for advice about eating a balanced diet.

For more information about food and nutrition, visit the U.S. Department of Agriculture Website at www.nutrition.gov or the American Dietetic Association Website at www.eatright.org.

H4. Hassle (Stress)

Most people's lives are very stressful at one time or another, but not everybody loses hair during these stressful episodes. This is because people's bodies react in different ways to stress. It seems that people who are more susceptible to stress induced hair loss are the ones who are more susceptible to hair loss in the first place. This means that stress is often only one of many factors influencing the hair cycle, rather than the only influence.

The hair can be affected by either an acute (severe) stressful episode, such as a sudden shock, or by a long-term stress situation. Obviously, you cannot avoid all stressful situations, so if your hair seems to be especially sensitive to stress, how can you deal with the problem?

Exercise

One of the best ways to reduce the effect of stress on your hair without taking medicine is to exercise. You should exercise at least three times a week for at least thirty minutes. When you are under more stress, increase your exercise frequency to five or six times a week. Any exercise that you enjoy should be adequate, as long as it increases your heart rate. Exercise has been shown to reduce anxiety, increase oxygen supply in the body, and reduce stress -related problems that can affect the hair cycle.

Relaxation And Meditation

Another way to help stress and hair loss is to relax or meditate (see References and Further Reading). A few minutes three to four times a week can really help to relieve stress. A good time to relax or meditate is after you have exercised, when you tend to be a little tired and can relax more easily (although don't fall asleep during relaxation or you will lose some of its benefits). Relaxing the mind helps your body relax and improves both physical and mental health. There are many different techniques you can try for relaxation, and I suggest using the one that best suits you. I have listed a few ideas just to get you started:

- **Deep breathing.** While sitting, take slow deep breaths and count to five as you inhale and five as you exhale. Repeat this three to five times.
- **Muscle relaxation.** While lying down, tense and then relax your arm and leg muscles one at a time. First, clench and then unclench

your fists one at a time, relaxing your arms on the floor. Second, lift and then lower your legs one at a time, leaving them relaxed on the floor. Lay relaxed for at least five minutes.

- **Music.** While sitting, listen to gentle music (preferably music without words). Music often helps soothe people's stress. Continue sitting for at least five minutes.
- **Bath.** Lie in a warm bath for a few minutes. It often helps to relax your body's muscles and can also help ease your anxiety.
- **Positive Thoughts.** Try to think of positive life events rather than dwelling on negative ones. Try to concentrate on something positive you did today or something you are looking forward to doing. Ignore any negative thoughts that may 'try' to enter your mind.

Talking to Someone

I find that it helps to talk to someone close to you about your hair anxieties. Often discussing your concerns about losing or thinning hair helps to diminish the stress that hair loss can cause. If you don't have someone close whom you can talk to, consider talking to a psychologist or trained hair specialist.

For more information about how to deal with stress, visit the American Psychological Association Website at www.apa.org, the Anxiety Disorders Association of America Website at www.adaa.org, or the International Stress Management Association Website at www.isma.org.uk.

H5. Healing (Medications)

If you are taking a medicine for a chronic illness or disease, then of course you must continue using it, even if it's causing hair loss. Your general health super-cedes your hair health.

However, if there are other treatments or medications for your illness, discuss with your physician the possibility of changing to another brand of medicine or another course of therapy. Remember that it may take three to six months before you notice that the treatment change is helping your hair.

If you find that the new treatment is not helping your hair-loss condition, then it may be due to one of the following:

- The disease itself is causing the hair problem.
- The medication type is causing the problem (meaning that all the medicines used to treat that type of condition can cause hair problems).
- Something other than the medicine is causing your hair to fall out.

H6. Hormones

I have discussed in H1. Hereditary some therapies that can be used for genetic hair loss, particularly ones that help reduce the activity of testosterone or dihydrotestosterone in the hair follicle. Also, in H5. Healing (in Chapter 3), I discussed that correcting your thyroid dosage will help control any hair loss from this particular problem.

For Men

Anabolic Steroids

Abusing anabolic steroids (synthetic versions of testosterone) can lead to hair loss. In Chapter 3, I described genetic hair loss as being caused by the conversion of testosterone to dihydrotestosterone (DHT). Therefore, in susceptible men these synthetic hormones can either trigger genetic hair loss or accelerate its progress.

For Women

Oral Contraceptive Pill

If you think the contraceptive pill that you are using may be causing hair loss, speak to your physician about changing the pill to one that contains a type of synthetic progesterone (*progestin*) with fewer male hormone side effects. Ones containing norgestimate (in Ortho-Cyclen, Ortho-Tri-Cyclen, and Ortho-Tri-Cyclen Lo), drospirenone (in Yasmin and Yaz), or ethynodiol diacetate (in Demulen, Zovia, and Kelnor) are purported to have less of these potential side effects.

Once you change the contraceptive pill, it may take three to six months for you to see if the new brand has helped improve your hair loss.

Polycystic Ovarian Syndrome

If you have been diagnosed with polycystic ovarian syndrome and you think it is causing your hair to fall out, ask your physician if you can take 100 to 200 milligrams of spironolactone per day with a contraceptive pill. As I mentioned in H1. Hereditary, this combination has been shown to help regrow hair in women with polycystic ovarian syndrome in small clinical trials (see References and Further Reading).

For more information about polycystic ovarian syndrome, visit the Polycystic Ovarian Syndrome Website at www.pcosupport.org.

Menopause

If you feel that menopause is causing your hair loss, speak to your physician about taking hormone replacement therapy or an over-the-counter herbal estrogen such as black cohosh or red clover.

For more information about menopause, visit the www.power-surge.com Website.

For Men and Women

Diabetes

This is a condition in which the body does not produce or properly use the hormone, insulin. This may cause many health problems including hair loss. Thus, having the condition diagnosed and treated as soon as possible is very important. Your physician should be able to confirm this condition through blood tests.

If the diabetes has affected your hair cycle, once your diabetes has been treated and brought under control, you should see improvement with your hair. Less will fall out and some regrowth should occur.

For more information about diabetes, visit the American Diabetes Association Website at www.diabetes.org, the Canadian Diabetes Association Website at www. diabetes.ca, or the Diabetes UK Website at www.diabetes.org.uk.

H7. Hairdressing

Improving your hair cosmetically is important even if you are using hair loss treatments or some of the lifestyle 7Hs to improve your hair. It is doubly important if all else has failed to arrest your hair loss or regrow your hair adequately. Therefore, this is an important component when dealing with hair loss, even though hair-loss specialists often do not discuss it. The bottom line for you in seeking help for your hair loss (and reading this book!) is that you want your hair to look good so that you have confidence when you step outside your home.

Within reason, I suggest you do what needs to be done to make your hair look presentable. For instance, if you color your hair and your roots are showing, then you should have the color done. When you are due for a color, you probably think that there is less hair on your head because the gray hair blends in with the scalp. Also, as gray hair is a loss of pigment (called melanin), the skin, which also contains this pigment, may lose some of its color as well, making the hair look thinner still. When you color your hair, make sure that you follow the instructions carefully (if done at home) or have it done professionally.

Also, if you have your hair straightened, you may need to continue doing this process; the area of hair that is between the virgin hair and relaxed hair tends to be very brittle and so is more likely to break.

If you have your hair permanently waved, the longer you wait between perms the flatter and thinner it will look, so continue to do these. Perms help swell the hair shaft and so give your hair more body, making it look fuller.

I suggest using a hair-strengthening treatment (there are many brands to choose from at your local pharmacy or cosmetic store) a week before and a week after any chemical processing to help strengthen the fiber. This will make it less susceptible to breakage after a chemical process has been carried out. Of course, if your hair has been overprocessed, then wait until the hair has been strengthened before doing another chemical process.

As mentioned in Chapter 3, if you brush your hair for styling, it is best to comb the tangles out first by combing from the ends to the roots. First, section your hair. Take an inch of the sectioned hair at the bottom, and comb out the tangles. Then move up to the next inch and comb downward. Keep doing this until that section of the hair has been detangled, and then move on to the next section. After you have combed out all the tangles, you can use a brush for styling

Regarding blow-drying, remember the motto: "If it's hurting the scalp, it's harming the hair". If you can feel the heat of the dryer on the scalp, then the temperature is too hot and you should turn it to a cooler temperature. A good idea is to test the heat of the dryer on your hand first. If it's too hot for your hand, it's too hot for your hair.

Wigs and Hairpieces

Sometimes, cosmetic improvement is not enough to make you comfortable with the way your hair looks. If this is the case, it may be wise to shop for a hairpiece,hair system, hair extensions, or a wig to help improve the appearance of your hair.

Hairpieces, hair extensions, and hair systems are often clipped or glued onto existing hair and are used to fill in a thin area of scalp or help lengthen the hair. Wigs usually cover the entire head and are often worn by people with very little or no hair (obviously, some people also wear wigs and hairpieces to instantly change their overall appearance). Many years ago, wigs and hairpieces appeared obvious and the wearer ended up being teased or mocked (usually behind his or her back). Nowadays, however, most wigs and hairpieces blend in extremely well with the existing hair and appear very natural. Some of my patients buy hairpieces and wigs while they wait for their treatment regimen to help regrow their hair.

Sometimes, however, wigs and hairpieces can be fitted poorly and lead to severe breakage (traction alopecia). Make sure that the person you are purchasing from is professional and has a good reputation (a friend's recommendation is helpful). As with finding a hair loss-specialist, it is best to do some homework first.

Hair Restoration and Hair Cloning

Hair restoration (also called hair-transplants) is another option for covering a thinning scalp or for filling-in your hair-line. I decided to get a hair transplant to help improve the overall density of my hair and found that it really complemented the hair growth that I had obtained from my own treatment regimen (see Preface). As with hairpieces and wigs, transplants were very noticeable many years ago. However, over the past decade or so they have become practically imperceptible.

With a hair transplant, a surgeon removes a donor area from the back of the scalp with the hair follicles intact and transplants these follicles into the thinning areas. It usually takes three to six months to notice a big improvement with hair growth, and many surgeons recommend using minoxidil, Propecia, and/or laser therapy to help with this regrowth. You can repeat the procedure many times to fill in other areas of the scalp that subsequently thin.

Before deciding on transplants, I suggest that you first find out why your hair is falling out. Some hair-loss conditions do not warrant a transplant because the hair will grow back anyway. Sometimes, the transplanted hair may also shed if the hair loss is because of telogen effluvium rather than genetic hair loss (see the Appendix for more information on these conditions).

Occasionally, a scalp reduction is used, where a piece of thinning scalp is completely removed and the surrounding hairy scalp is sewn back in place to fill in the area, either in conjunction with a transplant or instead of one.

Recently, hair cloning has been discussed in the press, although at the writing of this book, it is still some time away from being approved as a transplant option. The procedure for hair cloning is still being studied. However, it appears that one option is to first clone some hair follicle cells in a test tube or Petri dish and then carefully position these cells in the scalp. The placement of these cells encourages them to grow into a hair follicle and so produce a hair.

For more information about hair transplants and hair cloning, visit the International Society of Hair Restoration Surgery Web site at: www.ishrs.org.

Cover Crayons, Sprays, and Fibers

There are many different types of crayons, sprays, and fibers that are available to cosmetically help cover thinning areas. The crayons are used directly on the scalp to help hide thinning areas. The sprays and fibers are usually applied directly to the hair to add body and make the hair look fuller.

These options are used by many of my patients to good effect. They do not cause hair loss, though care should be taken when washing them out to reduce any potential hair breakage.

THE MULTI-TREATMENT APPROACH

I have suggested in this chapter that using a multi-treatment approach is the best way to treat a hair loss problem. Obviously, it depends on the causes of your hair loss to decide which are the best treatments. The more factors triggering your problem, the more treatment options you should use. Even if you have only one hair loss problem, such as, telogen effluvium (excessive hair shedding) or genetic hair loss, you should consider using a multi-treatment approach. This will increase your chances of improving your hair.

Sometimes, however, it may be too time consuming or costly to use the multi-treatment approach. In this case, choose a treatment regimen that you feel comfortable using, both in time it takes to apply and in its overall cost. Then continue using this treatment for at least three to six months to give it a chance to work. After this time, if you feel that it isn't working, stop using the original treatment and begin using a new treatment. Then give this new treatment three to six months to work.

If you feel a treatment is working but you need to change it due to its cost or it's too time consuming to apply, choose another treatment regimen. Instead of stopping the original treatment immediately, use *both* your previous and new treatments for three months before stopping the original treatment. This will allow the new treatment to take effect and reduce the possibility of hair shedding from stopping the original treatment.

THREE MONTHS? YOU'RE KIDDING!

It's easy for me (or any one else for that matter!) to tell you that the treatment regimen you have chosen needs at least three months to see whether it's working, but it's you who has to live with the worry for that period of time—and maybe longer. How can you do that? Many of my patients are beside themselves with concern and are often panicking that they are going bald. Every day seems a year, and every hair that falls seems to confirm the fear that they are going bald.

If you fall into this category and have not yet read Chapter 2, I suggest you do so. This chapter will help you cope with your condition on a daily basis while you are waiting for the treatment regimen to start working. It also gives you advice on how best to deal with the emotional problems often associated with hair loss.

I KNOW WHICH TREATMENT TO USE, HOW CAN I MONITOR IF IT'S WORKING?

So far you have ascertained whether you are losing your hair (Chapter 1). You are coping with the problem and not allowing it to affect your daily life (Chapter 2). You have determined, with the help of a hair-loss specialist, what is causing your hair loss (Chapter 3), and you've chosen a treatment regimen to help improve your condition (Chapter 4).

Now you need to wait at least three months to see whether the treatment is working. But how do you know whether it's *really* working and is not just wishful thinking? How can you monitor your hair-loss amount or size of a thinning area?

Chapter 5 discusses in detail several techniques you can use to more objectively tell whether your hair is improving or not. Like Chapter 2, this chapter is unique to hair-loss books because it systematically explains measuring techniques that you can do to see whether your hair is getting better (or not).

In short, Chapter 5 will help you decide whether the treatment you have chosen to use is working.

FIVE

HOW YOU CAN MONITOR WHETHER THE TREATMENT IS WORKING

You've decided on a treatment regimen. Now how do you know whether it's working? Basically, you want to see that new hair is growing, that there is a reduction in hair fall, and that you see less scalp, but how can you make an accurate assessment?

In this chapter I have put together many methods for you to use to monitor your own condition. Some are a little involved, while others are more straightforward. Use the ones you find that best serve your needs.

MONITORING HAIR LOSS BY USING GENETIC THINNING CHARTS

Monitoring Male Pattern Alopecia

To help you find the stage at which your hair loss has reached or to help you see whether you actually have a genetic hair loss pattern, review the following pictures that show eight of the stages of male pattern alopecia (there are other stages which have been omitted for simplicity). These stages were classified initially by J. B. Hamilton (1954) and then modified by O. T. Norwood (1975) (see References and Further Reading). This is one of the methods I use to monitor my patients' hair.

Although there are other scales to classify male pattern alopecia, dermatologists and trichologists most often use the Hamilton-Norwood scale to categorize type and extent of genetic hair loss in men. Hair-loss researchers also use this scale when studying hair loss treatments. The Hamilton-Norwood scale helps hair-loss experts worldwide have a common language when explaining treatment results in publications or diagnosing a particular patient's genetic hair loss. It enables them to keep track of the condition, that is, whether it is improving or worsening with or without treatments.

Classification of Male Pattern Alopecia

The following diagrams illustrate some of the stages of the Hamilton-Norwood classification for male pattern alopecia. You can use the Self-Classification Male Pattern Alopecia Chart (Table 5.1) to monitor the progress of your condition to see whether (and by how much) your hair is changing. This will be helpful if you are assessing the effectiveness of a particular treatment for your hair loss or if you are just watching for any possible changes in your hair quantity.

Table 5.1 will help you keep track of your male pattern alopecia condition. Note the date when you are assessing your hair loss in the left-hand column, and then look at the different Hamilton-Norwood stages to classify your own hair loss type. Put this in the right-hand column. You may find that your exact condition is not shown in any of the classifications, as it is impossible to include every hair-loss pattern. In this case, choose the stage that looks closest to your hair-loss type. Carefully look at each picture and read the notation to get a more accurate assessment of your particular condition.

Table 5.1: Self-Classification Male Pattern Alopecia Chart

Date	Hair-loss type

Type 1

Type 1 is also known as a "normal" adult male hair distribution, with no hair loss and very minimal frontal hairline or temple recession. Most men get a naturally higher hairline as they get older. This does not always mean that genetic hair loss is occurring.

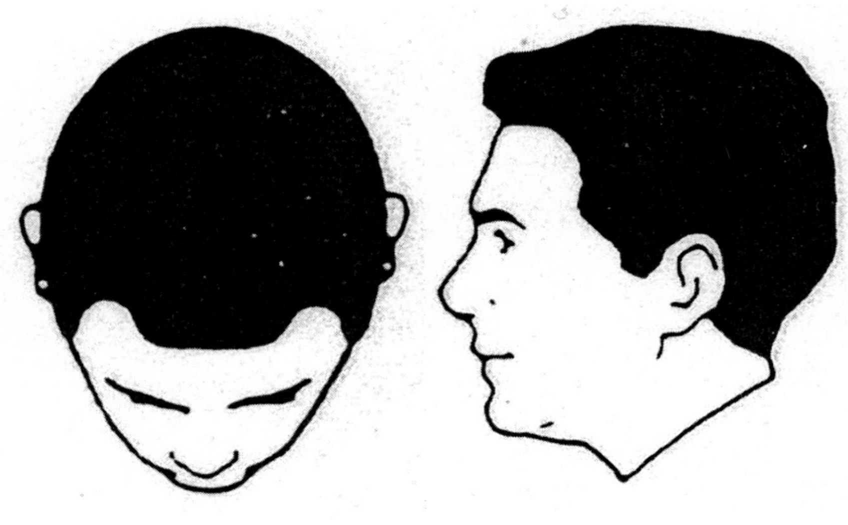

Type 1—Frontal View **Type 1—Side View**

Type 2

Type 2 is the first category that shows male pattern hair loss and is, therefore, the earliest stage. With this type, a mild or moderate recession at the temples has occurred. In the temple area, some finer, shorter hairs—some without pigment (called *vellus* hairs) —have replaced thicker, darker hairs (called *terminal* hairs). The crown area of the scalp has lost very little, if any, hair.

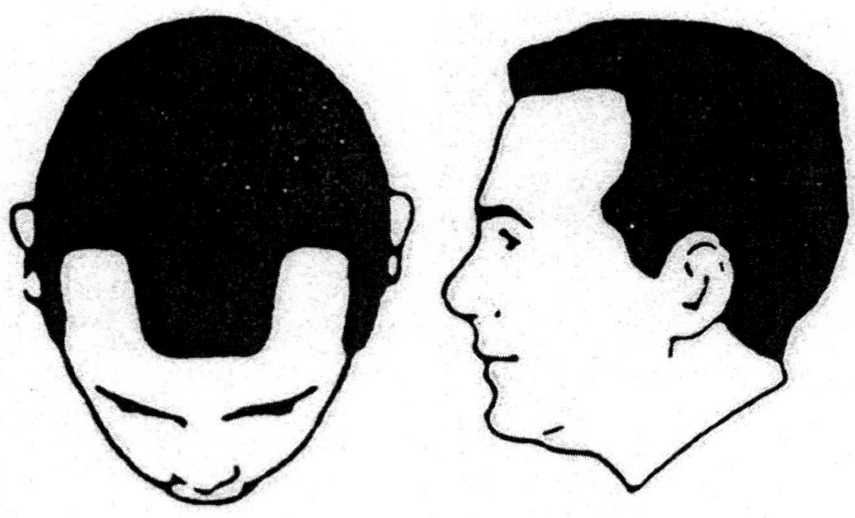

Type 2—Frontal View **Type 2—Side View**

Type 3

Type 3 is often regarded as the first stage of cosmetically apparent hair loss. Here the temples continue to recede. As with Type 2, vellus hairs replace the terminal hairs in the temple region. Very little hair loss has occurred on the crown area, although the mid-frontal area between the temples is beginning to thin.

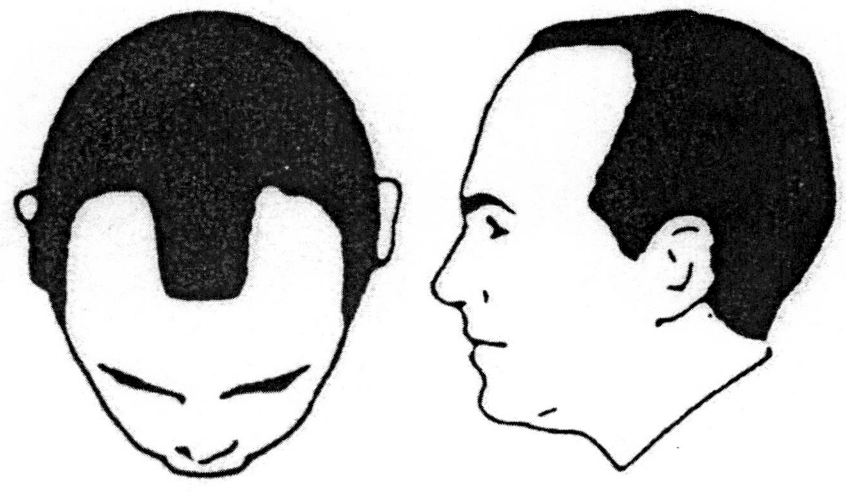

Type 3—Frontal View **Type 3—Side View**

Type 3-V

Type 3-V (*v* for "vertex" or "crown") is the stage where the temples have thinned in a similar fashion to Type 3; however, the crown hair is also starting to thin. The hair in the crown area is becoming shorter and finer, and the scalp is beginning to show through. Thinning in the mid-frontal area between the temples is also occurring.

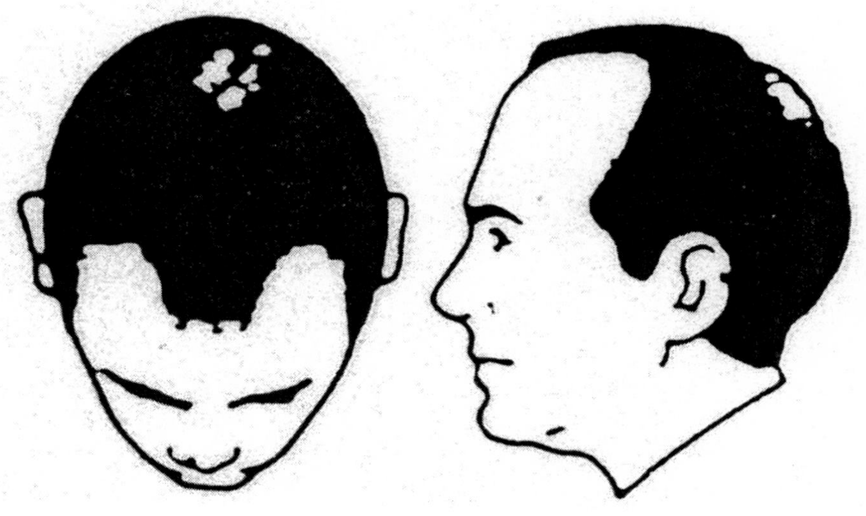

Type 3-V—Frontal View **Type 3-V—Side View**

Type 4

Type 4 shows the continued recession of the frontal and temple areas of the hairline, as well as the continued thinning of the crown area. The mid-frontal area of hair between the two temples is also continuing to thin, and the crown area of the scalp is more apparent. The hairs in the thinning areas are losing their pigment making the hair loss look more obvious.

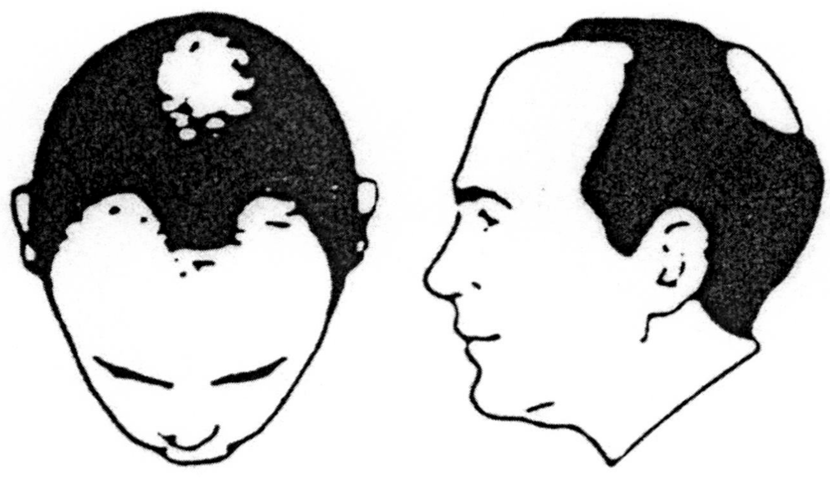

Type 4—Frontal View **Type 4—Side View**

Type 5

Type 5 is the combination of a more severe frontal recession and a greater degree of thinning to the crown area of the scalp. There is a general frontal recession in both the temple and mid-frontal areas that meets with the thinning crown area. The vellus hairs in all these areas are becoming even smaller and have taken on a downy appearance. In some cases, hair above the ears and along the neck hairline is beginning to recede.

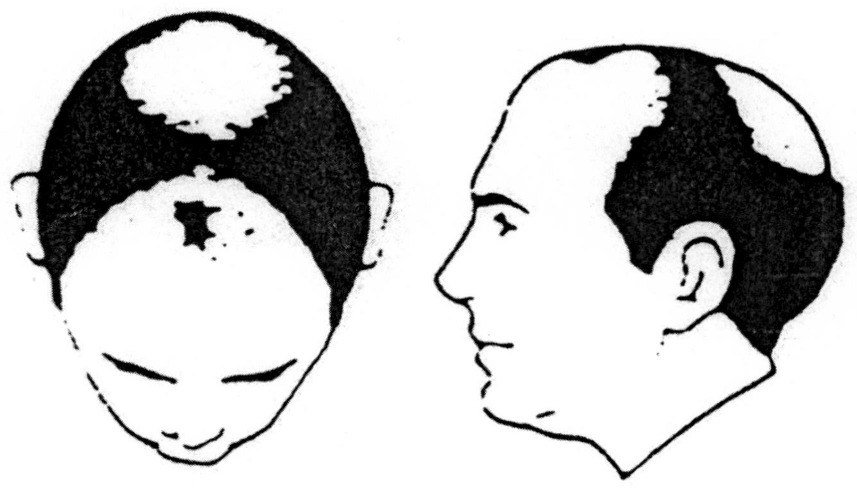

Type 5—Frontal View **Type 5—Side View**

Type 6

Type 6 shows a further worsening of both the mid-frontal, temple, and crown areas. These areas have very few terminal hairs, as most a re now vellus or downy hairs. If you are noticing hair loss above the ears or along the neck hairline, this too will worsen at this stage.

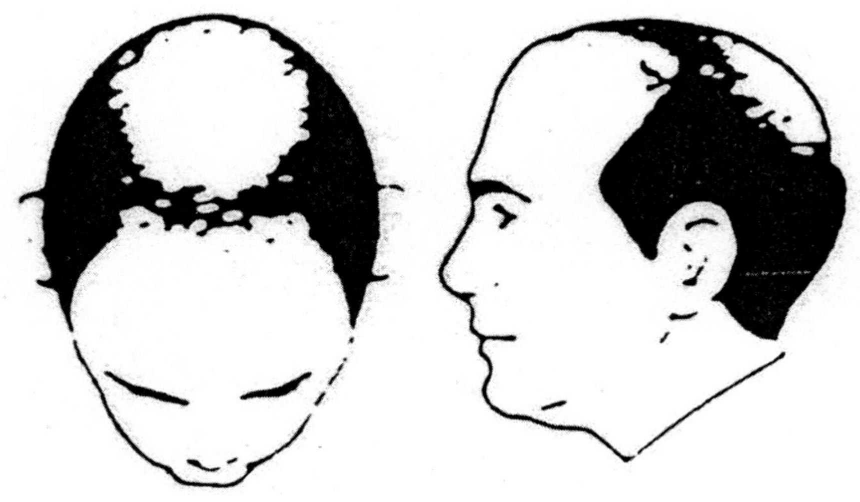

Type 6—Frontal View **Type 6—Side View**

Type 7

Type 7 is the most advanced classification of male pattern alopecia. Here the exi sting hair has been reduced to a horseshoe-shaped fringe on the sides and rear of the head. Only downy-looking vellus hairs are present on the crown or front areas, and most of these are too fine to see.

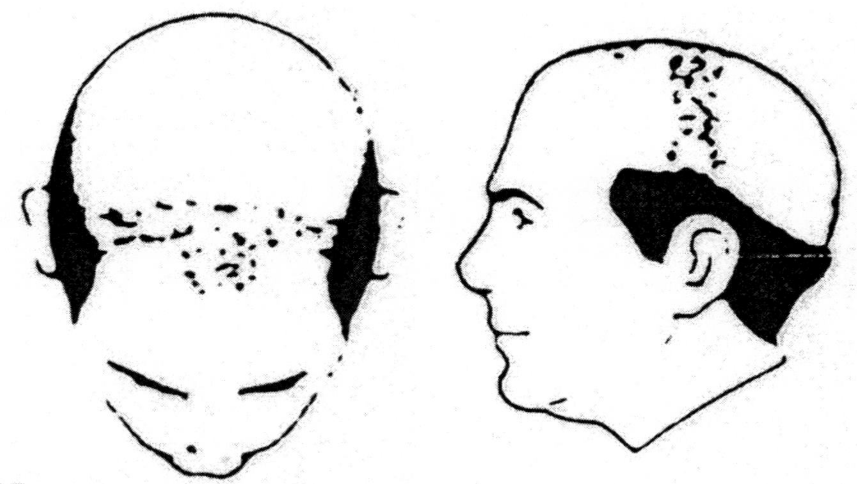

Type 7—Frontal View **Type 7—Side View**

When reassessing your hair loss after your initial classification, I suggest the minimum of a three-month gap between each assessment. In general, genetic changes can take a long time to occur.

Monitoring Female Pattern Hair Loss

E. Ludwig (1977) (see References and Further Reading) categorized female pattern hair loss into three grades. Although other classifications have been developed, as with the Hamilton scale for men, dermatologists, trichologists, and researchers most often use the Ludwig scale to categorize the type and extent of genetic hair loss in women. This is one of the methods I use to monitor my patients' hair.

Classification of Female Pattern Hair Loss

You may find that your exact condition is not shown in any of the classifications, particularly as there are only three stages. If this is the case, classify yourself into the nearest stage that looks closest to your hair-loss type. Carefully look at each picture and read each notation to get a more accurate assessment of your particular condition.

Use the Self-Classification Female Pattern Hair Loss Chart (Table 5. 2), to classify your hair-loss condition and to monitor its progress. This will help you assess the effectiveness of a particular treatment for your hair loss or help you watch for any possible changes taking place with your hair.

Note the date in the left-hand column and use the diagrams to classify your hair loss grade in the right-hand column of the table.

Table 5.2: Self Classification Female Pattern Hair Loss Chart

Date	Hair-loss grade

Grade 1

Grade 1 shows the early stages of female pattern hair loss. A mild thinning of the hair is occurring on the top and crown (fronto-vertex) areas of the scalp. Longer, thicker, darker hairs (called *terminal* hairs) are present, intermingled with some shorter, finer, less pigmented (*vellus*) hairs. The partings are beginning to get wider, but a well-preserved frontal fringe of hair is usually present.

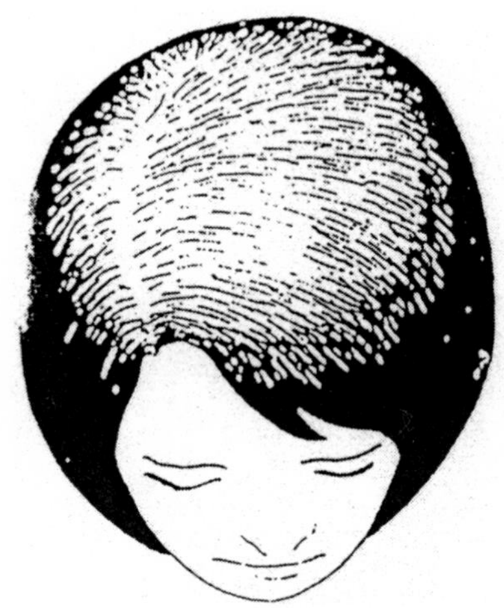

Grade 1—Frontal View

Grade 2

Grade 2 shows an advanced stage of female pattern hair loss. A pronounced thinning of the hair on the top and crown areas of the scalp occurs. The partings become wider, which makes the scalp more apparent, and more downy-looking hair (vellus) is present in between the longer, terminal hairs. A well-preserved frontal fringe is still present.

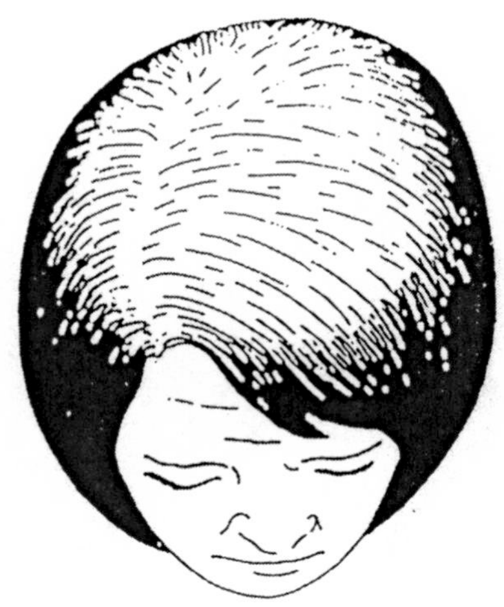

Grade 2—Frontal View

Grade 3

Grade 3 shows the final stage of female pattern hair loss. Almost total hair loss from the top and crown areas of the scalp has occurred. Many vellus hairs are present, with comparatively few terminal hairs. The frontal fringe of hair is smaller.

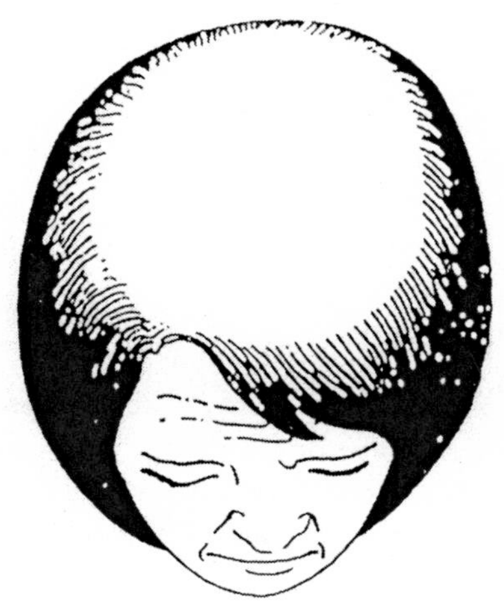

Grade 3—Frontal View

When reassessing your hair loss after your initial classification, I suggest the minimum of a three-month gap between each assessment. Genetic hair changes can take a long time to evolve.

MONITORING HAIR LOSS BY SIZE OF THINNING AREAS (FOR BOTH GENETIC AND NON-GENETIC HAIR LOSS)

Let's say that you want to measure whether the size of your thinning area is becoming wider. Possibly your temples are receding, the thinning spot on the crown of your head seems to be continuing to thin, and/or your partings are getting wider. You might also be using a hair-loss treatment and you want to see whether the thinning areas are regrowing.

How can you accurately measure whether your hair is thinning or regrowing? Which techniques are practical for you to do? This part of Chapter 5 explains some methods that you can use to accurately measure any changes (both positive and negative) that may be occurring with your hair.

Measure Using Photographs

A technique that you may find straightforward is photographing the area of hair either with a regular camera or digital one connected to your computer. With this technique, you can then measure the size of the thin area from the computer screen or from the photograph. This is one of the methods I use to chart the progress of my patients.

When taking photographs, it is important to note the amount of light that you use, the angle of your head, and when you last colored your hair (where relevant). This will enable you to compare your results with more confidence on subsequent measurements. Especially if you color your hair, it is important to make sure that the same length of time has passed from your last color, as gray or light hair will look thinner at the scalp level than colored or darker hair.

Follow these steps to take an overview picture.

1. Rest your chin snugly in your hands.
2. Pin the hair away from the area (if necessary) and take two or three pictures.
3. For the overview picture, make sure that you note the position of the camera and the distance it is from the scalp for future photographs.

Follow these steps to take pictures of different regions of the scalp.

1. With your mind's eye, divide the head into four regions: the right side, left side, top, and back.
2. When photographing the right side, use the right ear as the center of the photograph.

3. When photographing the left side, use the left ear as the center of the photograph.
4. When photographing the top of the head, use the midpoint between the crown and frontal hairline as the center of the picture.
5. When photographing the back of the head, use the point between the nape (the small indentation situated at the back of the head where it meets the top of the neck) and the crown as being the center of the photograph.
6. For future photographs, make sure that you note the position of the camera and the distance it is from the scalp.

After you have developed the pictures, simply measure the size of the thinning areas with a ruler. Over time you will be able to measure whether a thinning area is getting smaller or larger in size.

Measure Directly from the Scalp

A different technique that you could use is to actually measure the areas that you are concerned about directly from your scalp. For this you will need a measuring tape made from a substance that will lie flat on the contours of your scalp, such as paper. A wooden or flexible plastic ruler will not be accurate.

Make Your Own Ruler

If you do not have a measuring tape, you can easily make your own paper ruler from a photocopy. Use the metric side; it's easier to count in the tens of metric units than to convert parts of an inch with eighths and sixteenths. Also, you can more easily use decimals or count in either millimeters or centimeters. Use a transparent ruler to photocopy, as a solid ruler (such as one made from wood or metal) will not copy properly. Although the photocopying machine will not copy the ruler exactly on a 1:1 ratio, as long as you use the same ruler for each measurement, this won't be a problem.

Make sure the numbers of the side you are going to use to measure the area are clearly shown and that the millimeter graduations, which are the nine small lines between the centimeter numbers, are also clear. Do not photocopy both sides of the ruler—that is, both the metric and inch sides—as the paper ruler will be too wide and cumbersome. When cut, the paper ruler should only be about 3/4 inch (or 2 centimeters) in width.

If the ruler is too short, such as when you are measuring the crown, tape two rulers together or carefully note where the ruler ends and begin measurement with the same ruler from that exact spot.

How Often You Should Measure

The first time, take numerous measurements so that you can use the results as a basis for future comparisons. Then approximately every three months measure the area(s) again. As I mentioned in Chapter 4, it takes at least three and usually up to six months for you to see whether any changes are occurring due to treatments. Obviously, if you are losing hair rapidly, the thinning area may become larger more quickly and so more frequent measurements may be necessary. However, measuring too frequently may be counterproductive and lead you to obsess about your hair. Some of my patients count their hair or measure their thinning areas incessantly. I'm not saying that they shouldn't worry; however, looking to see whether your partings are wider every day is comparable to sitting on your porch each morning to watch the grass grow.

How to Measure

The following explanation outlines the best way to measure each part of your head. Of course, if you are only concerned about one part then just read about that area. In fact, all the methods are similar, and you can even introduce your own ideas to make the measuring easier. As long as you use the same technique each time, your method will be fine. If you are measuring without help from another person, it may be helpful to use a mirror to see that you are positioning the ruler correctly.

To Measure Hairline Recession

1. Run an invisible line with your mind's eye down the center of your head. The centerline of your head runs from the bridge of your nose to your nape (the small indentation situated at the back of the head where it meets the top of the neck).
2. Using the bridge of your nose (where the nose and forehead meet) as a starting point, simply measure the distance to the hairline at the center of your head.
3. Make a note of the measurement in Table 5.3: Measuring Hairline Recession.
4. Note the date of your measurement in the "Date" column of the table.

Table 5.3: Measuring Hairline Recession

Date	Distance from bridge of nose

To Measure Temple Recession

For your temples, use the same technique as with hairline recession but turn the ruler at an angle. I suggest using the furthest recession point because this area is likely to be the most actively receding.

1. For the measurement of your left temple recession from the bridge of your nose, put the distance in the "Left Temple: bridge of nose" column of the Table 5.4: Measuring Temple Recession.
2. For the measurement of your right temple recession from the bridge of your nose, put the distance in the "Right Temple: bridge of nose" column of the table.
3. To get a more accurate position of the receding area with a cross reading, put the ruler behind your ear on the side that you are measuring (where the ear attaches to the head at the position where glasses would sit), and note the distance to the receded temple.
4. For the measurement of your left temple recession from your left ear, put the distance in the "Left Temple: left ear" column of the table; and from your right ear, put the measurement in the "Right Temple: right ear" column.
5. Note the date of your measurements in the "Date" column of Table 5.4.

Table 5.4: Measuring Temple Recession

Date	Left Temple: bridge of nose	Left Temple: left ear	Right Temple: bridge of nose	Right Temple: right ear

To Measure an Area of Thinning on the Top or Crown Area

You can ascertain the size of a thin region on the top or crown of your head by simply measuring the diameter of that area. As the area is usually an irregular shape, I advise taking at least three measurements.

1. Using a paper measuring tape, first measure the largest part of the thin area (put this distance in the "Area: Largest" column of Table 5.5: Measuring Size of Thin Hair Region).
2. Measure the smallest part of the thin area (put this distance in the "Area: Smallest" column of the table).
3. Finally, measure what appears to be a middle-size part (put this distance in the "Area: Middle" column).
4. Note the date of your measurements in the "Date" column.

Table 5.5: Measuring Size of Thin Hair Region

Date	Area: Largest	Area: Smallest	Area: Middle

For a cross-reference, measure the distance between the edges of the thinning area from four positions of your head.

1. Use behind both your ears (where the ear attaches to the head at the position where glasses would sit) for the two side markers.
2. Use the bridge of the nose for the front marker.
3. Use the nape of your neck for a rear marker.
4. Enter the distance of the left ear from the left edge of the thin region in the "Area: from left ear" column of Table 5.6: Measuring Position of Thin Hair Region.
5. Enter the distance of the right ear from the right edge of the thin region in the "Area: from right ear" column of the table.
6. Enter the distance of the bridge of nose from the front edge of the thin region in the "Area: from bridge of nose" column.
7. Finally, enter the distance of the nape of neck from the rear edge of the thin region in the "Area: from nape of neck" column.
8. Note the date of your measurements in the "Date" column.

Table 5.6: Measuring Position of Thin Hair Region

Date	Area: from left ear	Area: from right ear	Area: from bridge of nose	Area: from nape of neck

If multiple thin areas are present, then use this technique for each individual area.

MONITORING HAIR LOSS BY COUNTING HAIRS THAT HAVE FALLEN OUT

Some of my patients tell me that they are continually running their fingers through their hair to see if any is coming out. If none falls on the first tug, then they repeat the process until they do see fall and think, "There, it's still falling out!" Others count the hair every day. If they have a day with a low hair count, they are ecstatic, thinking their hair fall has stopped; however, if they count a lot of hair, their day is miserable and nothing seems to go right. Are they being fair to themselves and their hair? Probably not. The amount of hair that they see will depend on many factors mentioned in previous chapters, such as when they washed or combed their hair previously (the longer between washes, the more hair they are likely to see due to accumulation). Hair growth is cyclical, so theoretically, we should shed the same number of hairs every day throughout the period of the cycle. However, just as the things that affect our body change each day, such as stress levels, different foods, and amount of exercise, the amount of hair that we lose will also differ on a daily basis.

The hair shedding that you are experiencing, therefore, may be nothing more than a normal occurrence. It is not so much the amount of hair you lose in one day that is important; it is the amount you are losing over a period of two or more weeks. If over that period of time your average hair shedding has increased drastically, you may be suffering from excessive hair loss.

So what would be a more accurate counting technique, one that would be more representative of your actual loss? I suggest that you simply count the hairs that are falling out during the wash. This will give a good indication as to whether the hair shedding is getting better or worse.

To use this method, it is best *not* to count the hairs on the comb or on the pillow because it increases your chances of inaccuracies (the more variables you have for collecting your sample, the more chance you have making an error). You can do this counting technique every week, every other week, or on a monthly basis. I often have my patients use this technique to self-monitor their hair loss.

Why Count The Hairs?

My patients use this technique most often. Most feel it makes them more active in their treatment, and many seem to enjoy it—especially if the numbers improve! Additionally, patients may experience hair-loss episodes between visits to my trichology centers that have subsided by the time I see them again (similar to the adage of going to a dentist with a toothache and, when getting there, forgetting which tooth hurts). This provides them with a quantitative assessment to give me for my comments and it enables me to closely assess how their hair is responding to treatment, especially as I may see them infrequently.

In-Office Hair Count

Counting hairs in-office can be a useful method for a hair-loss specialist to see how much hair loss a patient is experiencing.

Samples from Patients

Occasionally, patients bring their hair samples that they collected at home to my office; and my staff counts them. They count the number in the sample and divide by the number of days between hair washes. The result gives me a good indication to the quantity of hair that is falling out.

Pull Technique

At other times, I take my own sample with the "Pull Technique". This is a counting technique carried out at some hair-specialist offices (it was mentioned previously in Chapter 3 under the "Hair Pull Test" heading). It involves gently pulling small areas of hair to ascertain the amount of hairs that are in the telogen (resting) phase (these hairs will generally be the ones that will come out). These hairs can then be assessed. If there are a lot of hairs present after the hair has been pulled, it can give an idea of the excessive nature of the loss.

This technique is best done by a specialist and is not practical for self-monitoring your hair loss.

Method Of Self-Counting Hairs

To begin, each time you collect a hair sample, carefully comb your hair to remove any tangles and loose hair between thirty minutes and an hour before washing. Also, make sure that you have an empty hair catcher in the shower or sink drain when you wash your hair. Then wash your hair as normal. After you have finished, pick out the hair from the drain catch, put it in a tissue, and let it dry for a few hours. When it has dried, pick up the hair mass from the tissue and carefully count. You'll probably find it easier to see the smaller hairs if you use a white surface such as a countertop or piece of paper.

To help you do this counting technique, I have put an example in Table 5.7: Hair Wash Counting. You should carry out this technique over four consecutive washes, although only use three of the samples to work out your average hair loss. It is important to note the date of the wash before you collect the samples because the amount of hairs you see in the first wash sample will depend on when your hair was previously washed. As I pointed out in Chapter 1, the longer the time between washes, the more hair you will expect to lose. Therefore, washing your hair one, two, three, or more days before the first wash sample will determine how many hairs you count, and so following this pre-sample procedure is important. Collecting less than three samples tends to give inaccurate results and taking more than three samples is too time-consuming.

When you have counted your three samples, add them up for a total and then work out your daily average using Table 5.7. To get an accurate daily average, divide the hair sample total by the number of days between washes (see the "Explanation of Counting Hair" procedure following Table 5.7 for the best way to count your hair sample).

Table 5.7: Hair Wash Counting

Week Number	Pre-sample Date	First Wash		Second Wash		Third Wash		Total Hair Wash Amount (1 + 2 + 3) (A)	Total Number of Days (B)	Average Hair Wash Amount (A ÷ B)}
		Date	Hair Amount (1)	Date	Hair Amount (2)	Date	Hair Amount (3)			
Example	***1-Mar***	***2-Mar***	***35***	***3-Mar***	***50***	***5-Mar***	***95***	***180***	***4***	***45***
One										
Two										
Three										
Four										

Explanation of Counting Hair

Week One (Remember, you should take the samples over three consecutive washes.)

1. Note the date of the wash *before* you start collecting your hair samples. Put this date in the "Pre-sample Date" column.
2. The *next* time you wash your hair, note the date of this first wash in the "First Wash: Date" column.
3. Comb your hair between thirty minutes and an hour before washing.
4. Make sure that the hair catch is in the drain and cleaned of hair.
5. Shampoo and condition your hair as usual. Finish showering and then collect the hair in the hair catch.
6. Put the hair in a tissue, and allow it to dry for a few hours.
7. When dry, count the hairs carefully on a white surface. Put your total in the "First Wash: Hair Amount (1)" column.
8. The *next* time you wash your hair, note the date of this second wash in the "Second Wash: Date" column.
9. Repeat steps 3 to 6.
10. Put the total from the second wash in the "Second Wash: Hair Amount (2)" column.
11. The *next* time you wash your hair, note the date of this third wash in the "Third Wash: Date" column.
12. Repeat steps 3 to 6.
13. Put the total from the third wash in the "Third Wash: Hair Amount (3)" column.
14. Add the number of hairs from each of the three washes, and enter the total in the "Total Hair Wash Amount: 1 + 2 + 3 (A)" column.
15. Count the number of days between the pre-sample date and the date of the third wash (do not include the actual pre-sample date, but

do include the third wash date). Enter the number in the "Total Number of Days (B)" column.

16. Divide the total number of hairs (column A) by the number of days (column B). Put the result in the "Average Hair Wash Amount (A ÷ B)" column.

17. Repeat this procedure periodically, such as once a week or once a month. Put the next set of numbers in the row titled "Week Number: Two" and then "Week Number: Three", and so on.

Example 1 (From Table 5.7)

The date of the hair wash before my patient Lucy took her first hair sample was *March 1st,* which she entered in the "Pre-sample Date" column. The next day, Lucy took her first hair sample. She combed her hair thirty minutes before washing and made sure the hair catch was clean. She entered the date of this first wash (*March 2nd*) in the "First Wash: Date" column. When she had finished showering, she collected the hair sample from the drain catch, let it dry, and counted the hair. Then she entered the amount of *35* hairs in the "First Wash: Hair Amount (1)" column.

Lucy then washed her hair once more the next day. Before she started, again she combed her hair thirty minutes before washing and cleaned out the hair catch. She entered the date of this second wash (*March 3rd*) in the "Second Wash: Date" column. After collecting and counting this sample, Lucy entered the amount of *50* hairs in the "Second Wash: Hair Amount (2)" column.

Lucy was unable to wash her hair the next day, so she washed it the day after. She noted the date of this third wash (*March 5th*) in the "Third Wash: Date" column. Again, she cleaned the hair catch on the drain and combed her hair forty-five minutes before washing. She counted the hair sample from the drain catch and entered the total (*95*) in the "Third Wash: Hair Amount (3)" column. (As mentioned earlier, it is common for there to be an accumulation of hair loss the less often you wash your hair).

Next, Lucy added the number of hairs from each of the three washes (1 + 2 + 3) and entered the total (*180*) in the "Total Hair Wash Amount (A)" column. Then she counted the number of days between the pre-sample date and the date of the third wash. The pre-sample date was March 1st and the third was March 5th which, not counting the actual pre-sample date, is *4* days. She entered that number in the "Total Number of Days (B)" column.

Finally, Lucy worked out her average hair loss for that period by dividing column A by column B and getting *45* that she entered in the "Average Hair

Wash Amount (A ÷ B)" column. She kept this information to compare with future samples, the results of which she entered in the rows titled "Week Number: Two", "Week Number: Three", and so on.

What Do Your Results Mean?

What do your average hair wash results mean? Is your hair count high or normal? As I discussed in Chapter 1, for some people losing 40 hairs a day in the wash is normal, while for others it can be 120 hairs per day. Without doing a count when your hair loss is normal (which would be particularly unlikely as why would you even think of counting your hair if you're not worried about it falling out?), it is difficult to know what a normal count should be for you individually. Obviously, if your hair is thinning or you can see an excessive amount of hair strands all over the house or on your clothes, you can tell that the hair loss is high. Still you don't know if and when the shedding has returned to "normal".

Unfortunately, there is no easy answer. If you notice that your hair shedding has returned to a pre-hair-loss level or that your hair has stopped thinning or is actually improving, then the count should represent 'normal' quantities. In my experience, however, once people are worried about losing their hair, they are not objective when it comes to seeing that the loss has slowed. I suggest that you keep taking weekly or monthly counts until the number of hairs has dropped into the 40 to 120 window (plus or minus 10 to 15 hairs) and stabilized for three successive months. Of course, if you find that 120 hairs is too high a number for you individually, you'll want to make sure that your hair count s drop to an average of between 40 and 80 hairs. When the hair-loss amount seems to have remained the same for a few months, take a hair count every three to six months to make sure it has stabilized.

Total Daily Hair-Loss Average

How can you work out what your *total* daily hair loss is, not just the amount you lose in the wash? For you mathematicians (or for people handy with a calculator), you can do a simple calculation. I mentioned earlier that the amount of hair you lose in the wash represents about 75 to 80 percent of the total that you would expect to lose during the day (let's say it represents 80 percent). Use Table 5.8: Daily Hair Loss. Take your "Average Hair Wash Amount" total from Table 5.7: Hair Wash Counting and enter it in the "Average Hair Wash Amount (A)" column of Table 5.8. Divide this number by 4, and then multiply it by 5.

For example, Lucy entered her average hair wash amount of 45 hairs in the relevant box in Table 5.8. She also entered the date of when she calculated this average. She divided this number (A) by 4 and got 11.25 as her answer (B). Then she multiplied 11.25 by 5 to get a "Total Daily Hair Loss Average" of 56.25 or, rounding the number down, 56.

Doing this calculation will increase your expected normal hair loss average from between 40 and 120 hairs (the wash average) to between 50 and 150 per day. Some people feel that the amount of hair they lose during their wash represents a lower percentage than my example. While this may be true in some situations, I feel that 75 to 80 percent is the average if you consider normal washing and styling procedures.

Table 5.8: Daily Hair Loss

Week Number	Date	Average Hair Wash Amount (A)	Divide A By 4 (B)	Multiply B by 5	Total Daily Hair Loss Average
Example	5-Mar	45	11.25	56.25	56
One					
Two					
Three					
Four					

MEASURING HAIR GROWTH

Is your hair growing at the average speed? Do some areas grow a little slower than usual or not grow at all? Is the treatment you're using helping the hair grow faster or longer? One way to answer these questions is to measure your hair length over time.

As your hair grows at approximately 1/2 inch (1.2 centimeters) per month, working out whether it has grown in length should be a relatively straightforward way to monitor any improvement. Using your paper ruler, simply measure the length of hair in different areas of your head. Because hair tends to grow at a slightly different rate in different places on your head (which is why the hairs from different parts of your head are at different lengths before each trim, even if they were cut to the same length previously), it is best to take measurements from different areas.

Shortly after a trim or cut, measure the hair from the root to the tips in the following areas (note the measurements on Table 5.9: Measuring Hair Growth):

1. Mid-area between the crown and the nape (put the measurement in the "Between Crown & Nape" column).
2. At the crown of the head (put the measurement in the "Crown" column).
3. At the midpoint between the crown and frontal hairline (put the measurement in the "Between Crown & Hairline" column).
4. At the midpoint between the left ear and crown (put the measurement in the "Between Left Ear & Crown" column).
5. At the mid point between the right ear and crown (put the measurement in the "Between Right Ear & Crown" column).

Table 5.9: Measuring Hair Growth

Date	Between Crown & Nape	Crown	Between Crown & Hairline	Between Left Ear & Crown	Between Right Ear & Crown

If you color your hair, you can just measure how much the roots have grown in each of these areas.

I suggest re-measuring each area every one to three months to see whether there has been any hair growth.

As suggested at the beginning of this chapter, whichever measuring technique you decide to use, make sure the procedures you follow are consistent every time to ensure the most accurate measurements.

CONCLUSION

The Hair-Loss Cure: A Self-Help Guide has helped you to ascertain whether you are losing hair (Chapter 1) and has empowered you to not let the concern of losing your hair affect your quality of life (Chapter 2). It has also helped you to find out why your hair is falling out (Chapter 3), decide on a treatment regimen (Chapter 4), and evaluate the effectiveness of that treatment regimen (Chapter 5).

Chapter 6 helps bring all these points together by summarizing the previous chapters.

SIX

THE BOTTOM LINE

Losing hair can not only be devastating for a person, but all the commercials you see on TV or hear on the radio can make the situation even more difficult. When people begin to notice their hair falling out, they tend to panic and not think straight. They buy anything and everything that they see advertised, with little thought to what these products do or whether they will work for their particular hair-loss condition. Then, if the product or treatment doesn't work immediately, they will try something else until they have either exhausted all their options or spent all their money.

The bottom line to what you should do when you first notice your hair falling or thinning is to think about a strategy that makes the most sense to you and try to stick with it. Take control of your hair loss; don't let it control you.

I have five suggestions for you to follow that may help you form a plan of action:

1. Don't Panic!

I understand the worry that hair loss causes and the frustration that comes from trying to find the right treatment. This is why I advise you to take a step back and rationalize your condition, even though it may be hard. It is important that you don't panic and do the wrong thing.

If your hair loss is beginning to affect your mood and change your regular schedule, read Chapter 2 to help you cope.

2. Find Out *Why* You Are Losing Your Hair.

Seek a specialist who seems to know what he or she is doing, and make sure you are tested for all the most common causes of hair loss, such as thyroid problems, anemia or iron deficiency (especially in women), and so forth. Even if genetic hair loss is the most obvious reason, other factors that could be contributing to your hair loss or making it worse should be explored.

Even if you find two or more causes for your hair loss, each may not be playing an equal role. For instance, it could be that 90 percent of your hair loss is genetic, while only 10 percent is say, diet. Although a specialist is unable to give exact percentages to each cause, it is still worth understanding and finding all the contributing factors, however minor they may be.

To find out the reasons why your hair may be falling out, read Chapter3.

3. Treat *Each* of the Causes of Your Hair Loss.

Once the causes of your hair loss have been ascertained, try and correct what can be corrected, even if it only may be playing a very small role in your hair loss. For instance, taking the example I gave in the previous paragraph, if your poor diet is contributing only a small part to your hair loss, it should still be addressed. It may give you a better chance of seeing some improvement to your hair. I invariably suggest a multi-treatment approach to hair loss, as the more things you do, the faster and more likely you are to see results. Also, it makes you feel that something is being done and that you are being pro-active.

To help ascertain what the best treatments are for your hair-loss condition, read Chapter 4.

4. Be *Patient* Waiting for Your Treatment Regimen to Work.

This is often the most difficult thing to do, as you are losing hair and there appears no sign that the loss will stop. However, it often takes three months (sometimes up to six months) for a treatment to work. The more you change your treatment procedure before you have given it a fair chance, the more time and money you have wasted. If you are comfortable with the specialist and know that he or she has tried to find why your hair is falling out, then give that treatment program time before seeking other advice.

To monitor whether a treatment is working for you, read Chapter 5.

5. Don't be Afraid to Wash, Color, or Style Your Hair.

The importance of cosmetically improving your hair is often understated. As mentioned in previous chapters, the bottom line for you seeking treatments for your hair loss is so that when you look in the mirror, you feel comfortable with the way your hair looks. Within reason, do whatever you need to attain this sense of well-being.

OTHER GROUPS OF HAIR LOSS SUFFERERS

Not all people who are losing hair are worried and not all people who are worried about losing hair are actually losing it. These are two groups of people that are found on the opposite ends of the hair-loss spectrum. I have called them hair-loss contented and sufferers of hair dysmorphic disorder.

Hair-Loss Contented

If you've read this book, it probably means that you are losing hair and that you are worried. However, many men and women who are losing hair are not concerned at all. I call these people "non-motivated," meaning they are not motivated to search for professional help for their condition, because they are not distressed about losing hair.

I have done a large-scale study (see References and Further Reading) and found that people who say they are not bothered with losing hair are usually telling the truth. Furthermore, their hair-loss concerns compare favorably with people who have full heads of hair.

Groups such as "Bald is Beautiful" are content with their hair loss and have no motivation to seek treatment for their "condition" (see www.baldisbeautiful.org).

Hair Dysmorphic Disorder

In my experience, approximately 1 to 2 percent of people who complain of hair loss have no clinical signs of thinning hair other than normal day-to-day shedding (see References and Further Reading). I have labeled these people as ones with hair dysmorphic disorder (HDD).

Some people with HDD have other problems that they blame on their hair. These problems could be marital/family difficulties, job stress, and fear of getting older. They seem to focus their unhappiness on their hair, which leads them to feel that their hair is becoming thinner or falling out, when, in fact, it is not thinning at all.

Other people with HDD look at their hair in the mirror and get a distorted impression of its quantity, similar to people who look at their bodies and irrationally feel they are fat. These people look at their hair and think it is thinning or that they can see more scalp or that they used to have much more hair when, in fact, there is no change.

Additionally, there are people with HDD who did have a previous hair loss problem that has now grown back. However, they do not accept that their hair is better, and still feel that their hair is falling out or thinning.

In these instances, I recommend a checkup with their physician to make sure they are physically healthy. I try to explain that their hair is not thinning, but I do not dismiss the worry. I monitor their hair's stability by taking photos of their hair at that time and then comparing the photos to ones taken a few months later. I also try to cosmetically improve their condition so that they feel better about their hair.

Unfortunately, many people with HDD are ignored or derided by their physicians or families, but they need reassurances like any one else that are concerned about a particular health problem.

IN CONCLUSION

The Hair-Loss Cure: A Self-Help Guide has shown you that ***there is hope***. It has discussed that once you find out *why* you are losing hair, you are on the way to helping improve or even curing your condition. This book has also revealed that there are not only many *successful* treatment options to help your condition, but there are also specialists available who can help you choose the right treatments. Additionally, it has helped you cope with your hair loss and suggested ways to monitor any improvement.

Remember that not all hair loss is permanent and that there are many treatments that can help your condition. **Don't give up!**

APPENDIX: IN DEPTH

This appendix is for those who wish to learn a little more about hair and/or hair loss. In this section, I have added more technical information to what I discussed in previous chapters. This section touches the surface and only discusses the more common hair-loss conditions (there are many hair-loss conditions not mentioned). Because knowledge is increasing and more and more research is being done, I suggest that you continually search the Internet or your local library (look for medical and dermatology journals) for more up-to-date and detailed information (also see References and Further Reading).

TYPES OF HAIR

There are two types of hair on our body as adults: *terminal* and *vellus* hair. The other type of hair found on humans, *lanugo*, is seen on fetuses or newborn babies.

Terminal Hair

Terminal hair is the coarser hair found mainly over the scalp and eyebrows. At puberty, the action of hormones on the body hair produces terminal hair under the arms and over the pubic regions of both sexes. In men, it also appears on the face and chest.

Vellus Hair

Vellus hair s are the fine, downy hair found all over the body, except on the soles of the feet or on the palms of the hands (we don't have hair follicles in these areas). Vellus hair can also be found in the nose, to filter some of the dust and pollution from the air; in the ears, to protect them from foreign bodies; and in the windpipe (trachea) to help remove pollutants from the lungs.

Lanugo Hair

This type of hair is found only on fetuses and newborn babies. Lanugo hair is usually shed before birth or within the first few months of infancy.

HAIR STRUCTURE

Hair is made mostly of proteins, which account for about 85 to 90 percent of its structure. The main type of protein in the hair is called *keratin,* which is made up of small building blocks called amino acids, in particular cysteine, cystine, glutamic acid, and serine. The remaining 10 percent or so of the hair fiber is made up of *melanin* (the pigment that gives your hair its color), fats and oils, and water. The two main hair pigments are *phaeomelanin*, a yellow/red pigment that gives you red, blonde, or auburn hair, and *eumelanin*, a pigment that produces black or brown hair.

The hair shaft contains three layers, though sometimes only two if it is very fine. The outside layer is called the *cuticle*. Under a microscope, this looks like thin, flat scales placed one upon another, similar to slates on a roof. When these lift up and get caught in each other, the hair tangles. The middle, which is the largest part of the fiber, is called the *cortex* and looks like coils of ropes situated side by side. These help give the hair its relative strength. When the cortex is damaged, the hair becomes brittle and breaks easily. The inner part of the hair shaft (the layer that is often either not present or only partially complete) is shaped like a honeycomb and called the *medulla.* When present, the medulla can give a darker tinge to white hair, making it look gray.

The root of each hair is contained in a tube-like structure, called a *follicle*, which is situated approximately a quarter of an inch (6 millimeters) into the skin. Although it is part of the *epidermis* (outer layer of skin), the follicle extends through the *dermis* (middle layer of skin) into the *subcutaneous tissue* (inner layer of skin). The hair grows from the bottom of the follicle and is connected to a tissue structure called the *papilla*, which is nourished by a system of blood vessels. The cells of the papilla reproduce and move up the hair follicle, causing the hair to grow. Before these living cells reach the scalp surface, they lose moisture, harden, and die (a process known as *keratinization*) and subsequently become the hair fiber. This part of the hair fiber that you see appear from the scalp is a nonliving tissue that doesn't contain nerves (which is why having our hair cut doesn't hurt) or blood vessels (which is the reason we don't bleed when our hair is cut). A root sheath or covering at the base of the hair follicle helps anchor the hair fiber into the scalp, which is why your hair doesn't fall out when it is gently pulled.

A very small muscle, the *arrector pili* muscle, is attached to each follicle. When it contracts, the hair "stands on end," creating goose-bumps. Each follicle also has an oil gland attached (known as a *sebaceous gland*), which produces an oily secretion called *sebum*. Sebum is responsible for the oily "T-zone" on the forehead and around the sides of the nose, for some acne problems, and for certain dandruff conditions. At puberty there is an increase in oil production from our skin as the sebaceous glands become larger and increase their activity.

THE HAIR CYCLE

Hair growth is cyclical. The hair grows, goes through a transition stage, rests, and then falls out. Sometimes the follicle will enter a latent stage before the whole process begins again.

Anagen (the Growing Phase)

The growing phase has six stages, but the only one you see is the final stage, when the hair emerges from the scalp. Obviously, the longer your hair is in this phase the longer it will grow and the less you will see falling out. Also, your hair length will be determined by the speed of growth, which is, on average, 1.2 centimeters (1/2 inch) per month. The proportion of hair normally in this phase is 80 to 95 percent. Disruptions to the hair cycle during anagen are the main causes of hair loss.

Catagen (the Transition Phase)

The catagen or transition phase is the point where the hair has stopped growing and the root sheath, which anchors the hair into the follicle, begins to break down. The proportion of hair in this phase is less than 2 percent. This phase is rather insignificant as the hair is either growing (an anagen hair) or isn't (a resting hair). For this reason, most researchers will count catagen hairs (if they can find them!) in with telogen hairs.

Telogen (the Resting Phase)

During the telogen phase, the once-living cells near the bottom of the follicle (called the *papilla*) become hardened (*keratinized*) and form a club or bulb-type end. The follicle shrinks away from the papilla and eventually releases the hair (this shedding of the hair is sometimes called the *exogen phase).* The percentage of hair in the telogen phase is 5 to 18 percent. After about three months, the follicle will move back down to rejoin with the papilla and the whole cycle begins again.

With genetic hair loss, the follicle can go into a latent stage called the *kenogen* phase before restarting anagen.

AVERAGE DAILY HAIR LOSS

In Chapter 1, I mentioned the average daily hair loss should be about 40 to 120 hairs. How is this worked out?

If we put together the "for how long does my hair grow" and "how many hairs do I have on my head" information from Chapter 1, we can work out an average person's daily hair loss:

100,000 hairs (the average number of hairs)
divided by
1,000 days (the average hair cycle)
= 100 hairs/day

GENES

Genes are small portions of long, threadlike structures called *chromosomes.* Genes carry information to produce specific proteins. The action of chromosomes and genes are similar to a computer containing thousands of programs. For example, when you need a word processing program to write a letter, you activate it from the hard drive, which stores many different programs, and then you can produce the letter by typing. When you have finished using the program, you deactivate it. Similarly, when the body needs a certain protein (like a new hair), the relevant gene that is situated on a chromosome is turned "on" and 'expresses' itself. When the body has made enough of that particular protein, the gene is turned "off." It is believed that some hair-loss conditions are closely linked to this switching on and off of specific genes that control hair growth.

GENETIC HAIR LOSS

Genetic hair loss (men's genetic hair loss is called male pattern alopecia and women's is called female pattern hair loss) tends to affect a large majority of men and over half of women at some point in their lives (see References and Further Reading).

Causes of Genetic Hair Loss

Over the past 50 years or so, research into genetic hair loss has pointed to the genetic sensitivity to the male hormone dihydrotestosterone (DHT) as the main cause. The development of genetic hair loss is associated with the shortening of the anagen (growing) phase of the hair cycle and consequently with an increase in the proportion of telogen (resting) hairs. There is a reduction in the size of the affected follicles, which results in a reduction in the diameter of the hairs that they produce. This is an essential feature of this type of hair loss, which accounts for the thinning of the hair and the widening of the partings.

Male Pattern Alopecia

The onset of male pattern alopecia is linearly related to age; that is, 20 percent of men are experiencing some hair loss by age twenty; 30 percent of men are experiencing some hair loss by age thirty, and so on (see References and Further Reading).

The hair begins to recede at the temples and thin in the vertex (crown) area. Eventually, the whole fronto-vertex (between the hairline and crown) area of the scalp can be involved.

Female Pattern Hair Loss

Hair loss in women may be caused by another factor, in addition to DHT. Some recent research papers (see References and Further Reading) have suggested that a reduction in the activity or amount of an enzyme called *aromatase* (which converts certain male hormones in the scalp into female hormones) may also contribute to female pattern hair loss. This could account for the difference in clinical appearance between male pattern alopecia and female pattern hair loss, which is typically diffuse (evenly spread over the scalp) and affecting the frontal and vertex (crown) areas with similar severity. Often a band of slightly denser hair is retained along the frontal hairline.

Also, women can exhibit a normal amount of hair in the front area of their scalp, which gradually thins out as you look farther back near their crown. Called a "Christmas-tree" look, this is also indicative of a genetic condition. A male-type pattern of hair loss, marked by temple recession and/or complete thinning, is less frequent.

Treatments for Genetic Hair Loss

Treatments for genetic hair loss are discussed in Chapter 4: Treating Your Hair Loss (under H1. Heredity).

PATCHY HAIR LOSS (ALOPECIA AREATA)

Alopecia areata is characterized by patchy scalp hair loss and occasionally affects every hair follicle on the scalp (*alopecia totalis*) or body (*alopecia universalis*). The disease usually occurs between the ages of adolescence and thirty, but it can appear at any age and affects both sexes equally. Alopecia areata has a rapid onset but tends to spontaneously reverse.

Causes of Alopecia Areata

The causes of alopecia areata are unclear; however, its activation may be caused by one or more factors, such as genetics, autoimmune mechanisms, or environmental triggers such as stressful and emotional occurrences (see References and Further Reading).

Genetic Link

Some researchers theorize that there is a genetic link in a certain percentage of cases (some have suggested up to 20 percent), but this link is not as easy to identify as with genetic hair loss. This is because it is thought that many genes are responsible for alopecia areata (called *polygenic inheritance*) and all these genes need to be activated at the same time for the condition to develop. Because many genes need to be "in place" before the condition develops, alopecia areata can skip many generations before manifesting itself (see References and Further Reading).

Due to the possibility of a multi-gene influence on alopecia areata, it is difficult to pinpoint which family members, if any, are carriers of the genes responsible for the condition. However, if your alopecia areata condition does appear to be genetic, you will find that the severity of your condition will not necessarily follow that of the family member(s) who also suffer from the condition. This is due, in part, to the unpredictable nature of the condition. At the time this book was written, more research needs to be done to understand genetic influences on this condition.

Autoimmune Link

Alopecia areata is thought to be an autoimmune condition by some experts. They believe that the body's immune system attacks the hair follicles and disrupts the hair cycle due to a problem with the immune system's ability to distinguish between the "self" and "non-self" tissue.

Stress Link

Stress has long been thought by many experts to be a trigger for alopecia areata. As with the genetic and autoimmune links, stress' relevance to initiating the condition is not fully understood. Many researchers think that rather than stress causing alopecia areata, the condition is causing the stress, and so the stress is a byproduct rather than a cause.

Alopecia Areata Classification

The extent of hair loss from Alopecia Areata has been classified using the Severity of Alopecia Tool (SALT) into the following categories (see References and Further Reading):

S0: no hair loss
S1: less than 25 percent hair loss
S2: 25 to 49 percent hair loss
S3: 50 to 74 percent hair loss
S4a: 75 to 95 percent hair loss
S4b: 96 to 99 percent hair loss
S5: total scalp hair loss (alopecia totalis)
S5B2: total scalp and body hair loss (alopecia universalis)

Treatments for Alopecia Areata

Treatments for Alopecia Areata, used with varying success, include topical and systemic corticosteroids (including injecting steroids into the scalp), PUVA therapy (methoxypsolaren with ultra violet A), dinitrochlorobenzene (DNCB), squaric acid dibutyl ester, diphencyprone, nicotinic acid, an amino acid called tyrosine, and hypnotherapy.

For more information on alopecia areata, visit the National Alopecia Areata Foundation (NAAF) Website at: www.naaf.org

HAIR PULLING (TRICHOTILLOMANIA)

Trichotillomania is the loss or damage of scalp hair through repeated pulling or twisting due to irresistible compulsive impulses. It tends to be chronic and causes severe discomfort and social problems. It is classified as a "disturbance of impulse control" by the Diagnostic and Statistical Manual of Mental Disorders (see References and Further Reading) and is generally categorized with obsessive-compulsive disorders.

Trichotillomania is more common among children than adults and occurs more than twice as frequently in women than in men. It sometimes occurs with bulimia nervosa in teenage girls. The clinical feature of trichotillomania is plucked hair from the side of the fronto-parietal (between the hairline and crown) region of the scalp favoring the dominant hand. Occasionally, the whole scalp is affected. In rare cases, other body sites are involved, such as eyelashes, eyebrows, pubic hair, and perianal hair.

In some cases the hair can be chewed, eaten, and swallowed; this is called *trichophagy.*

Causes of Trichotillomania

The causes cited for trichotillomania depend upon which psychological discipline you refer to. Psychoanalysts attribute the condition, in part, to disruptions in psychosexual development, repressed aggression, and emotional deprivation during youth. Behaviorists compare the condition to other habits, such as thumb sucking and nail biting.

Trichotillomania does not have a genetic connection. Rather there is more likely to be an emotional cause, as with many psychological conditions, through the relationship between the person with trichotillomania and his or her parents. For instance, some researchers have found there to be a correlation particularly between girls with trichotillomania and problems, conscious or unconscious, with their mothers. Also, some studies have shown children pulling their hair from an area of their head in a similar position to where their father was experiencing male pattern alopecia (see References and Further Research).

Treatment for Trichotillomania

Behavioral modification through hypnotherapy and aversion therapy, psychotherapy, and prescription medicines are treatments used with varying degrees of success.

For more information on trichotillomania, visit the Trichotillomania Learning Center Website at: www.trich.org.

HAIR SHEDDING (TELOGEN EFFLUVIUM)

Also known as temporary hair loss, telogen effluvium is characterized by the anagen (growing) hairs prematurely entering the telogen (resting) phase of the hair cycle. Telogen effluvium usually presents itself as excessive shedding (also called *acute* TE). However, it can also manifest itself with a normal amount of hair loss leading to gradual thinning (also called *chronic* TE). With chronic TE, care needs to be taken to differentiate it from genetic hair loss. The hair fiber s in chronic TE usually do not become finer, as they do with hereditary thinning.

Causes of Telogen Effluvium

Telogen effluvium is usually not a condition directly affected by hereditary factors. Instead, it occurs due to a disturbance to the hair cycle that causes the hair to fall out prematurely. These disturbances to the hair cycle could be from a multitude of reasons (see the 7**H**s in Chapter 3: Why You Are Losing Hair).

Treatment of Telogen Effluvium

Telogen effluvium, in the short term, is rarely permanent. Once the causes for the hair loss have been ascertained and corrected (see Chapter 4: Treating Your Hair Loss), the hair cycle should normalize and the hair usually re-grows back to its previous thickness.

In the long term, chronic TE can lead to permanent loss of hair. However, as with acute TE, some hair will regrow once the causes for the condition are corrected (see Chapter 4: Treating Your Hair Loss—under the 7**H**s).

HAIR BREAKAGE (TRACTION ALOPECIA)

Traction alopecia is the breakage of hair along its shaft. One of the most common causes of traction alopecia is the damage to or absence of the cuticle or outside layer of the hair. This can lead to a multitude of hair fiber problems such as breakage, knotting, splitting, and dullness.

Causes of Traction Alopecia

There are many causes of traction alopecia. For instance, the hair, sometimes already weakened by chemical applications, can be easily broken by friction or by tension. Prolonged tension could even induce follicular inflammatory changes, which may eventually lead to scarring. Traction alopecia can also be induced easily in people with genetic hair loss. This is because the telogen (resting) hairs, which make up a higher proportion of the total, are more readily extracted than anagen (growing) hairs.

Traction alopecia can be aggravated by vigorous brushing, blow-drying, or incorrect massage techniques. As traction alopecia is mostly caused by hair breakage, any genetic condition that causes structural defects to the hair shaft, so making the fiber weaker, can cause the hair to be more susceptible to fracture (see References and Further Reading).

Defects of the Hair Shaft That Can Cause Traction Alopecia

Structural defects of the hair shaft can cause significant cosmetic problems, or they may render the hair abnormally susceptible to injury by minor degrees of trauma (see References and Further Reading).

Trichorrhexis Nodosa

Trichorrhexis is a distinctive response of the hair shaft to injury. The cuticle cells become damaged due to chemical or physical trauma, which causes the cortical cells to splay out and form nodes. These nodes are usually very weak and allow for the hair to break easily at these points.

Trichoptilosis

Trichoptilosis describes the longitudinal splitting of the hair shaft. It is also called *split ends.* This condition is also caused by chemical or physical trauma.

Trichonodosis

Trichonodosis is the knotting of the hair. It can occur spontaneously or through styling mistakes. Breakage frequently occurs, especially as the knot is removed.

Other Hair Shaft Defects

Other, rarer inherited hair fiber defects can cause the hair to grow in a bead-like fashion (called *monilethrix*); can cause the hair to have a twisted, corkscrew appearance (*pili torti); or can cause areas of the hair to lose their pigment and become very coarse and wiry over time (Menkes syndrome*). These conditions can weaken the hair shaft to such a degree that the hair will break easily enough to cause severe hair loss.

Treatments for Traction Alopecia

Treatments for traction alopecia are discussed in Chapter 4: Treating Your Hair Loss (under H7. Hairdressing).

SCARRING ALOPECIA

Scarring hair loss (also called *cicatricial alopecia*) is the generic term applied to alopecia that accompanies or follows the destruction of hair follicles, whether by a disease affecting the follicles themselves (primary cicatricial alopecia), or by some indirect process external to them (secondary cicatricial alopecia).

The skin often has a translucent ("onion skin") or depigmented look, sometimes accompanied by inflammation, and the hair loss can be patchy or diffuse. A biopsy is usually performed to identify the exact cause of this type of alopecia.

Examples of cicatricial alopecia are cutaneous lupus erythematosus, lichen planopilaris, and central centrifugal cicatricial alopecia.

Causes of Scarring Alopecia

The follicles may be absent as a result of a developmental defect, or they may be irretrievably injured by trauma, as with burns or continuous over-processing and pulling of the hair. They may also be destroyed by a specific and identifiable infection or by the encroachment of a benign or malignant tumor.

Treatment for Scarring Alopecia

Treatment for scarring alopecia is limited, as the condition is often permanent. However, systemic or topical corticosteroids are often used to reduce the inflammation and slow the progress of the disease (see References and Further Reading).

For more information on Scarring Alopecia, visit the Cicatricial Alopecia Research Foundation Website at: www.carfintl.org

THE PSYCHOLOGICAL IMPLICATIONS OF HAIR AND HAIR LOSS

As hair is very important for an individual's physical attractiveness (how others view you) and body image (how you view yourself), it follows that hair loss can affect a person's self-image, self-esteem, and overall quality of life (your everyday life and outlook). As a result, people who are losing their hair tend to become very worried about the consequences. Many cases have been reported of people becoming introverted and withdrawn due to the worry of losing their hair. This has been confirmed by research studies among men and women who are losing their hair (see References and Further Reading). Many participants reported that their lives had changed and their stress levels increased after they noticed a worsening of their hair quality or quantity—not before.

The manner in which people with genetic hair loss are affected by their condition is usually sex dependent. Women tend to be more ashamed, distressed, anxious and concerned about their hair loss; have lower self-esteem; and have more social problems than men with hair loss or women with normal amounts of hair. They also feel more uncomfortable in the presence of others. Studies of men with genetic hair loss are more conflicting. Some report minor social concerns but claim to maintain normal self-esteem and psychological profiles. Conversely, other studies have concluded that hair loss is indeed stressful to men, causing diminished feelings of attractiveness and social functioning; manifested by lower self-esteem and body image, and increased stress. These psychological effects seem to be influenced by a person's age, extent of hair loss, and marital status.

Hair-loss problems have also been described in both sexes as symptoms of other underlying psychological or personal problems (see References and Further Reading).

REFERENCES AND FURTHER READING

The following Websites, books, and medical journals were used as references in writing *The Hair-Loss Cure: A Self-Help Guide.*

I suggest that you look up some of these references if you wish to do further reading about a topic mentioned in this book. You can find many of these references online or in a local or university library. Obviously, there are numerous other resources and publications available to you. However, this comprehensive list should answer most of the questions that you may have.

WEBSITES

American Academy of Dermatologists	www.aad.org
American Diabetes Association	www.diabetes.org
American Dietetic Association	www.eatright.org
American Psychological Association	www.apa.org
Anxiety Disorders Association of America	www.adaa.org
Association of Psychocutaneous Medicine of North America	www.urmc.edu/derm/apmna/index.cfm
Bald Is Beautiful	www.baldisbeautiful.org
British Association of Dermatologists	www.bad.org.uk
British Science Corporation	www.HairAndScalp.com
Canadian Dermatology Association	www.dermatology.ca
Canadian Diabetes Association	www.diabetes.ca

Children's Alopecia Project	www.childrensalopecia project.org
Cicatricial Alopecia Research Foundation	www.carfintl.org
Diabetes UK	www.diabetes.org.uk
Dr. David H. Kingsley	www.DrDavidKingsley.com
European Hair Research Society	www.ehrs.org
Institute of Trichologists	www.trichologists.org.uk
International Association of Trichologists	www.trichology.edu.au
International Society for Quality of Life Research	www.isoqol.org
International Society of Hair Restoration Surgery	www.ishrs.org
International Stress Management Association	www.isma.org.uk
Menopause	www.WomensHealth.gov
National Alopecia Areata Foundation (NAAF)	www.naaf.org
North American Hair Research Society	www.nahrs.org
Patient-Reported Outcome and Quality of Life Instruments Database	www.proqolid.org
Polycystic Ovarian Syndrome	www.pcosupport.org
The Trichological Society	www.hairscientists.org
Trichotillomania Learning Center	www.trich.org
U.S. Department of Agriculture (food & nutritional advice)	www.nutrition.gov

BOOKS AND MEDICAL JOURNALS

American Psychiatric Association. *Diagnostic and Statistical Manual of Mental Disorders,* 4th ed. (DSM-IV-TR). Washington, D.C., 2000.

Berg C. *The Unconscious Significance of Hair.* Leicester: Blackfriars, 1951.

Buckwalter KC. The influence of skin disorders on sexual expression. *Sexuality and Disability,* 1982; 5(2): 98-106.

Bunker CB, Dowd PM. Alterations in scalp blood flow after the epicutaneous application of 3% minoxidil and 0.1% hexyl nicotinate in alopecia. *British Journal of Dermatology,* 1987; 117(5): 668-669.

Camacho F, Montagna W. *Trichology. Diseases of the Pilosebaceous Follicle.* Farmington: Karger Publishers. 1998.

Cash TF. Losing hair, losing points? The effects of male pattern baldness on social impression formation. *Journal of Applied Social Psychology*, 1990; 20(2): 154-167.

Cash TF. The psychological effects of androgenetic alopecia in men. *Journal of the American Academy of Dermatology*, 1992; 26: 926-931.

Cash TF, Price VH, Savin RC. Psychological effects of androgenetic alopecia on women: Comparisons with balding men and with female control subjects. *Journal of the American Academy of Dermatology, 1993; 29: 568-575.*

Cervia M, Rebora A. Age-related severity of male-pattern alopecia. *Dermatologica,* 1983; 166: 81-83.

Clayson DE, Maughan MR. Redheads and blonds: Stereotypic images. *Psychological Reports,* 1986; 59: 811-816.

Cooper W. *Hair: Sex, Society, Symbolism.* New York: Stein and Day, 1981.

Dawber R. *Diseases of the Hair and Scalp,* 3rd ed. Oxford: Blackwell Scientific Publications, 1997.

de Koning EB, Passchier J, Dekker FW. Psychological problems with hair loss in general practice and the treatment policies of general practitioners. *Psychological Report,* 1990; 67(3): 775-778.

Draelos ZD, Jacobson EL, Kim H, Kim M, Jacobson MK. A pilot study evaluating the efficacy of topically applied niacin derivatives for treatment of female pattern alopecia. *Journal of Cosmetic Dermatology,* 2006; 4(4): 258-259.

Eckert J. Diffuse hair loss in women: The psychopathology of those who complain. *Acta Psychiatrica Scandinavica*, 1976; 53(5): 321-327.

Franzoi SL, Anderson J, Frommelt S. Individual differences in men's perceptions of and reactions to thinning hair. *Journal of Social Psychology*, 1990; 130(2): 209

Friman PC, Finney JW, Christophersen ER. Behavioral treatment of trichotillomania: An evaluative review. *Behavior Therapy*, 1984; 15(3): 249-265.

Gosselin C. Hair loss, personality and attitudes. *Personality and Individual Differences*, 1984; 5(3): 365-369.

Hall JR, McGill JC. Hypnobehaviour treatment of self-destructive behaviour: Trichotillomania and bulimia in the same patient. *American Journal of Clinical Hypnosis*, 1986; 29(1): 39-46.

Hamilton JB. Patterned loss of hair in man: types and incidence. *Annals of the N.Y. Academy of Science, 1954; 53: 708-728.*

Hoedemaker C, van Egmond S, Sinclair R. Treatment of female pattern hair loss with a combination of spironolactone and minoxidil. *Australasian Journal of Dermatology*, 2007; 48 (1): 43-45.

Invernizzi G, Gala C, Russo R, Polenghi M, et al. Life events and personality factors in patients with alopecia areata. *Medical Science Research Psychology and Psychiatry*, 1987; 15(17-20): 1219-1220.

Kingsley DH. The development and validation of a quality of life measure for the impact of androgen-dependent alopecia. Ph.D thesis. Portsmouth University, Portsmouth; 1999.

Kingsley DH. A quality of life measure for the impact of androgen-dependent alopecia. *Quality of Life Research Journal.* 2000; 9 (3): 331.

Kingsley DH. The Kingsley Alopecia Profile (KAP). *The Compendium of Quality of Life Instruments*, Vol. 6. (2004).

Kingsley DH. The quality of life implications of androgenetic alopecia and the importance of helping patients deal with its psychological effects. Presented at the International Society of Hair Restoration Surgery, 12th Annual Meeting, Vancouver, Canada, August 11-15, 2004.

Kingsley DH. Hair Dysmorphic Disorder. Poster presentation at the Fifth International Congress of Hair Research, Vancouver, Canada, Jun 13-16, 2007.

Koblenzer CS. *Psychocutaneous Disease.* Orlando: Grune & Stratton, 1987.

Koblenzer CS. Stress and the skin. *Advances*, 1988; 5(4): 27-32.

Koo JYM, Do JH, Lee CS. Psychodermatology. *Journal of the American Academy of Dermatology*, 2000; 43: 848-853.

Lane JD, Seskevich JE, Pieper CF. Brief meditation training can improve perceived stress and negative mood. *Alternative Therapies*, 2007; 13(1): 38-44.

Ludwig E. Classification of the types of androgenetic alopecia (common baldness) occurring in the female sex. *British Journal of Dermatology*, 1977; 97: 247-254.

Maffei C, Fossati A, Rinaldi F, Riva E. Personality disorders and psychopathologic symptoms in patients with androgenetic alopecia. *Archives of Dermatology, 1994; 130(7): 868-872.*

Mauvais-Jarvis P, Vickers CF, Weplerre J (eds). *Percutaneous Absorption of Steroids.* New York: Academic Press, 1980.

Mercurio MG. Androgenetic Alopecia in Women: Diagnosis and Treatment. *Hospital Medicine,* 1997; 33(9): 30-38.

Mortimer CH, Rushton H, James KC. Effective medical treatment for common baldness in women. *Clinical and Experimental Dermatology,* 1984; 9: 342-350.

Norwood O. *Hair Transplant Surgery. Springfield,* Illinois: Charles C. Thomas, 1973.

Norwood O. Male pattern baldness: Classification and incidence. *Southern Medical Journal,* 1975; 68: 1359-1365.

Olsen EA, Weiner MS, DeLong ER, Pinnell SR. Topical minoxidil in early male pattern alopecia. *Journal of the American Academy of Dermatology,* 1985; 13: 185-192.

Olsen E. *Diseases of Hair Growth: Diagnosis and Treatment,* 2nd ed. McGraw-Hill, 2003.

Olsen EA, Hordinsky MK, Price VH, Roberts JL, Shapiro J, Canfield D, et al. Alopecia Areata investigational assessment guidelines—Part II. *Journal American Academy of Dermatology,* 2004; 51(3): 440-447.

Olsen EA, Messenger AG, Shapiro J, et al. Evaluation and treatment of male and female pattern hair loss. *Journal of the American Academy of Dermatology*, 2005; 54(5): 301-311.

Olsen EA, Hordinsky MK, Whiting D, *et al.* The importance of dual 5 alpha-reductase inhibition in the treatment of male pattern hair loss: Results of a randomized placebo-controlled study of dutasteride versus finasteride. *Journal of the American Academy of Dermatology*, 2006; 55(6): 1014-1023.

Passchier J, Rijpma SE, Dutree-Meulenberg RO, Verhage F, et al. Why men with hair loss go to the doctor. *Psychological Reports,* 1989; 65(1): 323-330.

Passchier J, Van der Donk J, Dutree-Meulenberg ROGM, Stolz E, Verhage F. Psychological characteristics of men with alopecia androgenetica and effects of treatment with topical minoxidil: An exploratory study. *International Journal of Dematology,* 1988; 27(suppl.): 441-446.

Patzer GL. Psychologic and Sociologic Dimensions of Hair: An Aspect of the Physical Attractiveness Phenomenon. *Clinical Dermatology,* 1988; 6(4): 93-101.

Prager N, Bickett K, French N, Marcovici G. A randomized, double-blind, placebo-controlled trial to determine the effectiveness of botanically derived inhibitors of 5-alpha-reductase in the treatment of androgenetic alopecia. *Journal of Alternative and Complementary Medicine,* 2002; 8(2): 143-152.

Rittmaster RS. Finasteride. *New England Journal of Medicine,* 1994; 330: 120-125.

Robinson A, Jones W. Changes in scalp hair after cancer chemotherapy. *European Journal of Cancer and Clinical Oncology,* 1989; 25(1): 155-156.

Rogers NE, Avram MR. Medical treatments for male and female pattern hair loss. *Journal of the American Academy of Dermatology,* 2008; 59(4): 547-566.

Rook A, Dawber RPR. *Diseases of the Hair and Scalp*, 2nd ed. Blackwell, 1991.

Rook's Textbook of Dermatology, 7th ed. Blackwell, 2004.

Ross EK, Tan E, Shapiro J. Update on primary cicatricial alopecias. *Journal of the American Academy of Dermatology,* 2004; 53(1): 1-37.

Rushton DH, James KC, Mortimer CH. The unit area trichogram in the assessment of androgen-dependent alopecia. *British Journal of Dermatology,* 1983; 109: 429-437.

Rushton DH. Chemical and morphological properties of scalp hair in normal and abnormal states. Ph.D thesis. University of Wales, Cardiff; 1988.

Rushton DH, Ramsay ID, James KC, Norris MJ, Gilkes JJH. Biochemical and trichological characterisation of diffuse alopecia in women. *British Journal of Dermatology*, 1990; 123: 187-197.

Rushton DH, Futterweit W, Kingsley DH, et al. Quantitative assessment of spironolactone treatment in women with diffuse androgen-dependent alopecia. *Journal Society of Cosmetic Chemistry, 1991; 42: 317-325.*

Rushton DH, Ramsay ID. The importance of adequate serum ferritin levels during oral cyproterone acetate and ethinyl oestradiol treatment of diffuse androgen-dependent alopecia in women. *Clinical Endocrinology,* 1992; 36: 421-427.

Rushton DH, de Brouwer B, de Coster W, van Neste DJ. Comparative evaluation of scalp hair by phototrichogram and unit area trichogram analysis within the same subjects. *Acta Derm Venereol.* 1993 Apr; 73(2): 150-153.

Rushton DH, Dover R, Norris MJ, Gilkes JJH. Iron and hair loss in women; what is deficiency? This is the real question! *Journal of the American Academy of Dermatology,* 2007; 56(3): 518-519.

Satino JL, Markou M. Hair regrowth and increased hair tensile strength using the HairMax LaserComb for Low-Level Laser Therapy. *International Journal of Cosmetic Surgery and Aesthetic Dermatology,* 2003; 5 (2): 113-117.

Sawaya ME, Price VH. Different levels of 5alpha-reductase type I and II, aromatase, and androgen receptor in hair follicles of women and men with androgenetic alopecia. *Journal of Investigative Dermatology,* 1997: Sep; 109(3): 296-300.

Shum KW, Cullen DR, Messenger AG. Hair loss in women with hyperandrogenism: four cases responding to finasteride. *Journal of the American Academy of Dermatology,* 2002; 47: 733-739.

Sigelman L, Dawson E, Nitz M, Whicker ML. Hair loss and electability: The bald truth. *Journal of Nonverbal Behavior,* 1990; 14(4): 269-283.

Swedo SE, Leonard HL. Trichotillomania. An obsessive compulsive spectrum disorder? *Psychiatry Clinic North America,* 1992; 15(4): 777-790.

Thom E. Nourkrin®: Objective and Subjective Effects and Tolerability in Persons with Hair Loss. *Journal of International Medical Research,* 2006; 34: 514-519.

Toback C, Rajkumar S. The emotional disturbance underlying alopecia areata, alopecia totalis and trichotillomania. *Child Psychiatry and Human Development, 1979; 10(2): 114-117.*

Trost LB, Bergfeld WF, Calogeras E. The diagnosis and treatment of iron deficiency and its potential relationship to hair loss. *Journal of the American Academy of Dermatology,* 2006; 54(5): 824-844.

Uno H, Cappas A, Brigham P. Action of topical minoxidil in the bald stump-tailed macaque. *Journal of the American Academy of Dermatology,* 1987 Mar; 16(3 Pt 2): 657-668.

van der Donk J, Passchier J, Dutree-Meulenberg ROGM, Stolz E, Verhage F. Psychological characteristics of men with alopecia androgenetica and their modification. *International Journal of Dermatology,* 1991; 30(1): 22-28.

van der Donk J, Passchier J, Knegt-Junk C, Van der Wegen-Keijer MH, Nieboer C, Stolz E, Verhage F. Psychological characteristics of women with androgenetic alopecia: A controlled study. *British Journal of Dermatology,* 1991; 125: 248-252.

Van Neste DJ. Contrast enhanced phototrichogram (CE-PTG): an improved non-invasive technique for measurement of scalp hair dynamics in androgenetic alopecia—validation study with histology after transverse sectioning of scalp biopsies. *European Journal of Dermatology.* 2001: Jul-Aug; 11(4):326-331.

Venning VA, Dawber RP. Patterned androgenic alopecia in women. *Journal of the American Academy of Dermatology.* 1988 May;18(5 Pt 1): 1073-1077.

Walker SR & Rosser RM. *Quality of Life Assessment: Key Issues in the 1990's.* Lancaster: Kluwer Academic, 1993.

Wells PA, Willmoth T, Russell RJ. Does fortune favour the bald? Psychological correlates of hair loss in males. *British Journal of Psychology*, 1995; 86 (3): 337-344.

Whiting DA, Waldstreicher J, Sanchez M, Kaufman KD. Measuring reversal of hair miniaturization in androgenetic alopecia by follicular counts in horizontal sections of serial scalp biopsies: results of finasteride 1 mg treatment of men and postmenopausal women. *Journal of Investigative Dermatology*. 1999 Dec; 4 (3): 282-284.

INDEX

I

K

L

M

LaVergne, TN USA
17 January 2011
212791LV00006B/79/P

9 781935 278047